IASLC

INTERNATIONAL ASSOCIATION
FOR THE STUDY OF LUNG CANCER

Staging
Manual in
Thoracic Oncology

International Association for the Study of Lung Cancer
Denver, CO, USA

Executive Editor:
Peter Goldstraw, FRCS
Chair, IASLC Staging Project
Royal Brompton Hospital, Imperial College,
London, England

An IASLC publication published by Editorial Rx Press
Original cover and book layout design by Biographics

Editorial Rx Press, Registered Office:
P.O. Box 794,
Orange Park, FL, USA 32067
www.editorialrxpress.com

First Editorial Rx Press Printing July 2009
10 9 8 7 6 5 4 3 2 1

ISBN: 978-0-9799274-3-0

INTERNATIONAL ASSOCIATION
FOR THE STUDY OF LUNG CANCER

Staging
Manual in
Thoracic Oncology

Peter Goldstraw, FRCS, Executive Editor

2009

An International Association for the Study of Lung Cancer Publication

Editorial Rx Press
Orange Park, FL, USA

CONTENTS

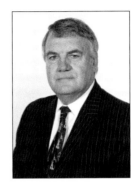

Peter Goldstraw, FRCS
Executive Editor

CONTRIBUTORS |

Editorial Committee

Peter Goldstraw (Chair, IASLC Staging Project), Royal Brompton Hospital, Imperial College, London, UK.

Hisao Asamura (Japan Lung Cancer Society Liaison) National Cancer Centre Hospital, Tokyo, Japan.

Paul Bunn (Board of Directors Liaison), Executive Director IASLC, University of Colorado Health Sciences, Denver, Colorado, USA.

John Crowley (Statistician), CEO, Cancer Research And Biostatistics, Seattle, Washington, USA.

James Jett (Editor, *Journal of Thoracic Oncology*), Mayo Clinic, Rochester, Minnesota, USA.

Ramon Rami-Porta (Vice-Chair, IASLC Staging Project), Hospital Universitario Mutua de Terrassa, Terrassa, Spain.

Valerie Rusch (American Joint Committee on Cancer Liaison). Memorial Sloan-Kettering Cancer Center, New York, New York, USA.

Leslie Sobin (International Union Against Cancer Liaison), Armed Forces Institute of Pathology, Washington, DC, USA.

On behalf of past and present members of the IASLC Staging Committee

IASLC International Staging Committee:

P. Goldstraw (Chairperson), Royal Brompton Hospital, Imperial College, London, UK; H. Asamura, National Cancer Centre Hospital, Tokyo, Japan; D. Ball, Peter MacCallum Cancer Centre, East Melbourne, Australia; V. Bolejack, Cancer Research And Biostatistics, Seattle, Washington, USA; E. Brambilla, Laboratoire de Pathologie Cellulaire, Grenoble, France; P. A. Bunn, University of Colorado Health Sciences, Denver, Colorado, USA; D. Carney, Mater Misericordiae Hospital, Dublin, Ireland; K. Chansky, Cancer Research And Biostatistics, Seattle, Washington, USA; T. Le Chevalier (resigned), Institute Gustave Roussy, Villejuif, France; J. Crowley, Cancer Research And Biostatistics, Seattle, Washington, USA; R. Ginsberg (deceased), Memorial Sloan-Kettering Cancer Center, New York, New York, USA; D. Giroux, Cancer Research And Biostatistics, Seattle, Washington, USA; P. Groome, Queen's Cancer Research Institute, Kingston, Ontario, Canada; H. H. Hansen (retired), National University Hospital, Copenhagen, Denmark; P. Van Houtte, Institute Jules Bordet, Bruxelles, Belgium; J.-G. Im (retired), Seoul National University Hospital, Seoul, South Korea; J. R. Jett, Mayo Clinic, Rochester, Minnesota, USA; H. Kato (retired), Tokyo Medical University, Tokyo, Japan; C. Kennedy, University of Sydney, Sydney, Australia; H. Kondo, Shizuoka Cancer Centre, Shizuoka, Japan; M. Krasnik, Gentofte Hospital, Copenhagen, Denmark; J. van Meerbeeck, University Hospital, Ghent, Belgium: T. Naruke (deceased), Saiseikai Central Hospital, Tokyo, Japan; H. Pass, New York Medical Centre, New York, New York, USA; E. F. Patz, Duke University Medical Center, Durham, North Carolina, USA; P. E. Postmus, Vrije Universiteit Medical Center, Amsterdam, the Netherlands; R. Rami-Porta, Hospital Universitario Mutua de Terrassa, Terrassa, Spain; V. Rusch, Memorial Sloan-Kettering Cancer Center, New York, New York, USA; N. Saijo, National Cancer Center Hospital East, Chiba, Japan; J. P. Sculier, Institute Jules Bordet, Bruxelles, Belgium; F. A. Shepherd, University of Toronto, Toronto, Ontario, Canada; Y. Shimosato (retired), National Cancer Centre, Tokyo, Japan; L. Sobin, Armed Forces Institute of Pathology, Washington, DC, USA; W. Travis, Memorial Sloan-Kettering Cancer Center, New York, New York, USA; M. Tsuboi, Tokyo Medical University, Tokyo, Japan; R. Tsuchiya (retired), National Cancer Centre, Tokyo, Japan; E. Vallieres, Swedish Cancer Institute, Seattle, Washington, USA; J. Vansteenkiste, Leuven Lung Cancer Group, Leuven, Belgium; H. Watanabe, National Cancer Centre Hospital, Tokyo, Japan; Y. Watanabe (deceased), Kanazawa Medical University, Uchinada, Japan; and H. Yokomise (retired), Kagawa University, Kagawa, Japan.

ACKNOWLEDGMENTS |

The IASLC would like to record its gratitude to our sponsors and the contributing databases: Eli Lilly and Company provided funding to support the International Association for the Study of Lung Cancer (IASLC) Staging Committee's work to establish a database and to suggest revisions to the sixth edition of the *TNM Classification of Malignant Tumours* through a restricted grant. Lilly had no input into the committee's analysis of the data or in their suggestions for revisions to the staging system.

The project was also supported by the AJCC grant "Improving AJCC/UICC TNM Cancer Staging."

Participating Institutions:
O. Visser, Amsterdam Cancer Registry, Amsterdam, The Netherlands; R. Tsuchiya and T. Naruke (deceased), Japanese Joint Committee of Lung Cancer Registry; J. P. Van Meerbeeck, Flemish Lung Cancer Registry-VRGT, Brussels, Belgium; H. Bülzebruck, Thorax-klinik am Universitatsklinikum, Heidelberg, Germany; R. Allison and L. Tripcony, Queensland Radium Institute, Herston, Australia; X. Wang, D. Watson, and J. Herndon, Cancer and Leukemia Group B (CALGB), Chicago, Illinois, USA; R. J. Stevens, Medical Research Council Clinical Trials Unit, London, England; A. Depierre, E. Quoix, and Q. Tran, Intergroupe Francophone de Cancerologie Thoracique (IFCT), Paris, France; J. R. Jett and S. Mandrekar, North Central Cancer Treatment Group (NCCTG), Rochester, Minnesota, USA; J. H. Schiller and R. J. Gray, Eastern Cooperative Oncology Group (ECOG), Boston, Massachusetts, USA; J. L. Duque-Medina

and A. Lopez-Encuentra, Bronchogenic Carcinoma Co-operative Group of the Spanish Society of Pneumology and Thoracic Surgery (GCCB-S), Spain; J. J. Crowley, Southwest Oncology Group (SWOG), Ann Arbor, Michigan, USA; J. J. Crowley and K. M. W. Pisters, Bimodality Lung Oncology Team (BLOT), USA; T. E. Strand, Cancer Registry of Norway, Oslo; S. Swann and H. Choy, Radiation Therapy Oncology Group (RTOG), Philadelphia, Pennsylvania, USA; R. Damhuis, Rotterdam Cancer Registry, Rotterdam, The Netherlands; R. Komaki and P. K. Allen, MD Anderson Cancer Center-Radiation Therapy (MDACC-RT), Houston, Texas, USA; J. P. Sculier and M. Paesmans, European Lung Cancer Working Party (ELCWP), Brussels, Belgium; Y. L. Wu, Guangdong Provincial People's Hospital, Guangzhou, People's Republic of China; M. Pesek and H. Krosnarova, Faculty Hospital Plzen, Plzen, Czech Republic; T. Le Chevalier and A. Dunant, International Adjuvant Lung Cancer Trial (IALT), Villejuif, France; B. McCaughan and C. Kennedy, University of Sydney, Sydney, Australia; F. Shepherd and M. Whitehead, National Cancer Institute of Canada (NCIC), Toronto, Ontario, Canada; J. Jassem and W. Ryzman, Medical University of Gdansk, Gdansk, Poland; G. V. Scagliotti and P. Borasio, Universita' Degli Studi di Torino, S Luigi Hospital, Orbassano, Italy; K. M. Fong and L. Passmore, Prince Charles Hospital, Brisbane, Australia; V. W. Rusch and B. J. Park, Memorial Sloan-Kettering Cancer Center, New York, New York, USA; H. J. Baek, Korea Cancer Centre Hospital, Seoul, South Korea; R. P. Perng, Taiwan Lung Cancer Society, Taiwan; R. C. Yung and A. Gramatikova, John Hopkins University, Baltimore, Maryland, USA; J. Vansteenkiste, Leuven Lung Cancer Group (LLCG), Leuven, Belgium; C. Brambilla and M. Colonna, Grenoble University Hospital-Isere Cancer Registry, Grenoble, France; J. Hunt and A. Park, Western Hospital, Melbourne, Australia; J. P. Sculier and T. Berghmans, Institute of Jules Bordet, Brussels, Belgium; A. K. Cangir, Ankara University School of Medicine, Ankara, Turkey; D. Subotic, Clinical Centre of Serbia, Belgrade, Serbia; R. Rosell and V. Aberola, Spanish Lung Cancer Group (SLCG), Spain; A. A. Vaporciyan and A. M. Correa, MD Anderson Cancer Center-Thoracic and Cardiovascular Surgery (MDACC-TCVS), Houston, Texas, USA; J. P. Pignon, T. Le Chevalier, and R. Komaki, Institut Gustave Roussy (IGR), Paris, France; T. Orlowski, Institute of Lung Diseases, Warsaw, Poland; D. Ball and J. Matthews, Peter MacCallum Cancer Institute, East Melbourne, Australia; M. Tsao, Princess Margaret Hospital, Toronto, Ontario, Canada; S. Darwish, Policlinic of Perugia, Perugia, Italy; H. I. Pass and T. Stevens, Karmanos Cancer Institute, Wayne State University, Detroit, Michigan, USA; G. Wright, St Vincent's Hospital, Victoria, Australia; C. Legrand and J. P. van Meerbeeck, European Organisation for Research and Treatment of Cancer (EORTC), Brussels, Belgium.

PREFACE

By Nagahiro Saijo, MD
IASLC President, 2007-2009

The International Association for the Study of Lung Cancer (IASLC) is proud to present the details of the IASLC/International Union Against Cancer (UICC)/ American Joint Committee on Cancer (AJCC) Revised Staging Classification for Lung Cancer in this Manual. The IASLC is the largest world-wide professional organization solely dedicated to reducing the worldwide burden of lung cancer. The International Staging Classification for Lung Cancer provides the basis for assigning prognosis and treatment selection for patients with lung cancer. Thus, its importance cannot be overemphasized, especially as we develop new methods of staging. These new methods include clinical procedures such as computed tomographic (CT) scans and CT/positron emission tomographic (PET) scans and new pathologic procedures such as endobronchial ultrasound (EBUS)-guided biopsies and video-assisted thoracic surgeon (VATS) biopsies. The IASLC recognizes that the staging classification will be most valuable and accurate if it is based on large numbers of cases carefully collected and analyzed. We are indebted to the diligent efforts of the IASLC Staging Committees chaired by Dr. Peter Goldstraw and whose members are listed in the Manual; the diligent efforts of the Cancer Research And Biostatistics (CRAB) office headed by Dr. John Crowley; the support of the IASLC Board of Directors whose members are also listed in the Manual; the financial support of Eli Lilly and Company and the support of the UICC and the AJCC to create a staging classification supported worldwide. We thank these individuals and organizations for their support and trust the revised staging classification will improve the outcome for lung cancer patients and their families.

INTRODUCTION

By Peter Goldstraw, FRCS, Executive Editor
Chair, IASLC Staging Project

With the release of the seventh edition of the *TNM Classification of Malignant Tumours*, the publication of this educational material represents the final phase of the work of the International Association for the Study of Lung Cancer (IASLC) Staging Committee for this revision cycle. The project has entailed an enormous amount of effort from past and present members of the committee, some of whom did not live to see the fruition of their work. We were indeed fortunate to develop a close working relationship with the dedicated and experienced team at Cancer Research And Biostatistics (CRAB). We are grateful to the International Union Against Cancer (UICC) and the American Joint Committee on Cancer (AJCC), who have collaborated and supported this initiative and provided much valuable advice; to Eli Lilly and Company, which generously provided the initial funding for this immense effort through an educational grant to the IASLC; and to the AJCC, who awarded funding for the additional work. We all owe an enormous debt of gratitude to those institutions and their patients, who provided that most precious commodity–their data. The work of all these parties, listed elsewhere in this book, has resulted in the largest database of lung tumors ever established to support the revision of the TNM classification, sourced from 46 databases in more than 20 countries around the world. A unique feature of this work has been the intensive validation, both internal and external, which should ensure that the proposals are appropriate to cases treated by all modalities of care and for patients seeking treatment around the world.

We hope that the new TNM classification will benefit patients worldwide, whatever the anatomical extent of their disease.

The IASLC books, produced in collaboration with the UICC and AJCC, are the first such site-specific guidelines on the TNM classification of thoracic malignancies. We hope that those involved in the research and care of patients with these diseases find them useful. We are grateful to the UICC and AJCC for permission to reproduce chapters that will appear in their own publications. Dr. Aletta Frazier brought to the project her experience as a radiologist and her skill as a medical artist. We thank her for the textural detail and accuracy of the resultant illustrations and her patience and persistence when faced with multiple revisions. Ms. Deb Whippen and her team at Editorial Rx, Inc., deserve our gratitude and admiration for the speed and precision with which these products were made available.

This is the first venture by the IASLC in this field, and we thank you for any suggestions you have as to how we can improve such material for the eighth edition of TNM, which is due in 2016.

Editor's Note: The editor's involvement with the IASLC Staging Project spans 13 years during which time he has gained some insight into the origins and development of the TNM classification for lung cancer, the important part played by a few far far-sighted and industrious individuals and the relationship between the two bodies that now administer the system worldwide, the UICC and AJCC. Through the good offices of Drs. Leslie Sobin, Brian O'Sullivan, and Thierry le Chevalier he has had access to the archives of the UICC and of the Institute Gustave Roussy. These archives are degrading and many important documents are already lost. It is hoped that this chapter will allow the reader to understand the motives that lead to the establishment of the IASLC Staging Project and to appreciate why this has proven to be such a milestone in the development of TNM, not only in lung cancer, but hopefully providing a template for similar initiatives in other organ sites.

CHAPTER 1 | The History of TNM Staging in Lung Cancer
–Peter Goldstraw

Efforts to develop an international language for the classification of cancer by describing the anatomical extent of disease started at the beginning of the 20th century.(1) During the first half of that century a number of organizations attempted to develop such systems and there were attempts to achieve an international consensus. From 1929 the lead was taken by the Radiological Sub-Commission of the Cancer Commission of the League of Nations Health Organization. They developed rules and definitions, created a classification by the anatomical extent of disease, identified the data elements required for the assessment of the results of treatment and went on to produce an Atlas, in 3 languages, showing the classification of cancer by stage. Although primarily concerned with carcinoma of the cervix these principles were widely accepted by other organizations. In 1950 three other organizations established committees to focus on this aspect of cancer: the World Health Organization Expert Committee on Health Statistics established its sub-committee on the Registration of Cases of Cancer as well as their Statistical Presentation, the 6th International Congress of Radiology created the International Commission on Stage-Grouping in Cancer and Presentation of the Results of Cancer (ICPR) and the Union Internationale Contre le Cancer (UICC) founded in Paris in 1934, now the International Union Against Cancer, established a Committee on Tumour Nomenclature and Statistics (CTNS).

During this period Professor Pierre Denoix (Figure 1.1), a surgeon at the Institut Gustave-Roussy in Paris, developed his system for the classi-

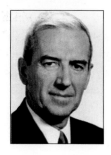

Figure 1.1 Dr. Pierre Denoix, 1912–1990. Surgical oncologist at the Institut Gustave-Roussy, Paris, Director of the Institut Gustave-Roussy 1956–1982. Chairman of the UICC Committee on Clinical Stage Classification and Applied Statistics, 1954–1966. President of the UICC 1973–1978. Commander of the Legion of Honour.

fication of malignant tumors, based upon "TNM," publishing a series of articles between 1943 and 1952 (2). He presented his "Uniform Technique for Clinical Classification by the TNM System" at the 7th International Congress of Radiology in 1953, and thereafter the ICPR adopted TNM as the basis of its classification for cancer of the larynx and breast. The next year the UICC replaced the CTNS with a special Committee on Clinical Stage Classification and Applied Statistics (CCSCAS) under the chairmanship of Professor Denoix. For the next 4 years this committee refined the general principles of TNM and undertook extensive international consultation on its proposals. The UICC then undertook a program to publish brochures or "fascicles" in which TNM classifications were proposed for cancer in different organ sites. In all, between 1960 and 1967, nine brochures were produced covering 23 sites, lung being included in a brochure published in 1966. The intention was to review the proposals for each site after a 5 year period of "field trials." In 1966 the UICC replaced the CCSCAS with a Committee of TNM Classification under the chairmanship of Mr. Michael Harmer. At this time the UICC was using both the French and Anglophone versions of its title, but gradually came to prefer the Anglicized form, while retaining the French abbreviation.

In 1968 the proposals contained in the brochures were brought together in the UICC "TNM Classification of Malignant Tumours,"(3) lung cancer being included under the section on "other sites." The T descriptors, in this first classification for lung cancer, included T0 for cases in which one could find no evidence of the primary tumor, T1 for tumors confined to a segmental bronchus or to a segment of one lobe, T2 in which tumor was confined to a lobar bronchus or one lobe, T3 in which tumor was involving the main bronchus or more than one lobe, and T4 for tumors extending beyond the lung. The N descriptors were NX, N0 and N1, in which there was "enlargement" of "intrathoracic" lymph nodes on "clinical, radiological or endoscopic evidence." These intrathoracic lymph nodes were further divided in to "hilar" or "peripheral" nodes, but as yet, there was no mention of nodes in the mediastinum. The M1 category was sub-divided into M1a, in which there was a pleural effusion with malignant cells, M1b cases with "palpable" cervical nodes and M1c for cases in which there were other distant metastases. Stage groupings were not proposed at this time and the classification was restricted to recording the anatomical extent of disease following clinical evaluation, subsequently designated as cTNM.

The American Joint Committee for Cancer Staging and End Results Reporting (AJC) was created in 1959, with representatives of the American College of Radiology, the American College of Surgeons, the College of American Pathologists, the American College of Physicians, the American Cancer Society and the National Cancer Institute. In 1980 it was renamed as the American Joint Committee on Cancer (AJCC). The AJC developed a separate and distinctive process from that of the UICC, employing "Task Forces" to gather data on specific cancer sites and to use this data to inform its proposals. The emergence of this new organization re-focused American participation away from the UICC and resulted in the possibility that these two organizations could make different, and possibly conflicting, recommendations to the cancer community. In 1968 there followed a series of meetings between the AJC and UICC and finally a "rapprochement" was reached, ensuring that neither would publish further recommendations without consultation with the other. In 1969 this agreement was extended to include "as far as practicable, other National TNM Committees and International non-governmental professional organizations."

In 1973 Drs. Mountain, Carr and Anderson reported the results of a study, undertaken under the auspices of the Task Force on Lung Cancer of the AJC, to develop "A Clinical Staging System for Lung Cancer."(4) Their proposals were derived from a data base of 2,155 cases of lung cancer, of which 1,712 were cases of non-small cell lung cancer (NSCLC), diagnosed at least 4 years before analysis. Practically all of the T descriptors in use today were introduced in that report, including the use of a 3 cm cut-off point for size, the impact on T category of invasion of the visceral and parietal pleura, the chest wall, diaphragm and mediastinum, the bronchoscopic criteria of T category and those based upon the extent of atelectasis or obstructive pneumonitis. The T categories proposed by the UICC were reduced with the loss of the T4 category, but an N2 category was added to address the issue of mediastinal node involvement. Malignant pleural effusion was reclassified from M1 to become a T3 descriptor. For the first time, the concept of stage groups was introduced, incorporating TNM subsets with similar prognoses "in a manner intended to minimize intragroup variability in survival and to create the greatest prognostic differences between stage groups." There were

18 possible permutations of the T, N, and M categories, grouped into stages I, II, and III. Four of the possible TNM sets had too few cases for analysis and 7 others contained less than 100 cases, 1 as few as 24. Stage I included T1 N0 M0, T2 N0 M0, and T1 N1 M0 subsets; Stage II accommodated T2 N1 M0 cases; and the other 14 TNM subsets all fell within Stage III. Graphs showed distinct differences in 5-year survival between each of the T, N, and M categories and the three stage groupings. A table showed different survival at 12 and 18 months for those TNM sets for which data were available, but no validation was presented for any of the individual descriptors. These proposals, although somewhat flawed in retrospect, represented the first attempt at data-driven revisions to the TNM classification of lung cancer. They were incorporated in to the 2nd edition of the UICC TNM Classification of Malignant Tumours published in 1975 (5) and the 1st edition of the Manual for Staging of Cancer published by the AJC in 1977.(6)

The 3rd edition of the UICC manual, published in 1978 (7) and enlarged and revised in 1982, was approved by National TNM committees in Canada, Germany, and Japan and the ICPR. In this edition, Stage I was further divided into Ia and Ib (N.B. at that time stage sub-groups were lower case) and stage IV was established for M1 disease. For the first time a separate classification was established to record the post-surgical histopathologic extent of disease (pTNM), and additional descriptors were introduced of "y" to identify classification performed during or following initial multimodality therapy and "r" for classification of recurrent tumors after a disease-free interval, and the optional use of the "C" factor was allowed to reflect the validity of classification according to the diagnostic methods employed. The Americans, however, were still using the previous classification which was published, without change, as the 2nd edition of their manual in 1983,(8) now under the auspices of the AJCC.

In 1986 Dr. Mountain (Figure 1.2) published "A new International Staging System for Lung Cancer"(9) based upon his own database which, at that time, contained 3,753 cases of lung cancer with a minimum follow-up of 2 years. His proposals were widely discussed at meetings held in 1985 between the AJCC, the UICC, and cancer committees from Germany and Japan, and when

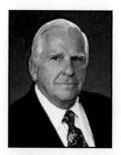

Figure 1.2 Dr. Clifton Fletcher Mountain, 1924–2007. Thoracic Surgeon, Chief of Thoracic Surgery, Chair of Surgical Department, MD Anderson 1960–1996. Founding member of the IASLC 1973, and President 1977.

accepted, once more brought in to line the classification of lung cancer in 4th edition of the UICC manual, published in 1987 (10) and the 3rd edition of the American manual published in 1988. (11) The changes that now came in to force included the classification of superficial tumors in which invasion was limited to the bronchial wall as T1 irrespective of location, the recommendation that the occasional pleural effusion that was cytologically negative could be ignored in defining the T category, the re-emergence of the T4 category and the creation of an N3 category. The existing T3 descriptors were split between the T3 category and the new T4 category on the basis that the former would retain those tumors that were "candidates for complete resection" while the latter category would contain tumors which were considered to be "inoperable." The previous descriptor of "mediastinal invasion" was split into its component parts, with invasion of the mediastinal pleura or pericardium remaining T3 descriptors while invasion of the great vessels, heart, trachea, oesophagus, carina and vertebral bodies became T4 descriptors, along with the presence of a pleural effusion. The situation was confused by the additional definitions of the T3 and T4 categories given in the text. Those tumors with "limited, circumscribed extrapulmonary extension" were to be retained within the T3 category while those with "extensive extrapulmonary extension" now fell in to the new T4 category. These conflicting definitions caused some confusion. Were tumors invading such structures as the pericardium still classified as T3 even if there was extensive invasion and they were considered inoperable? Or, in such circumstances did they become T4? If invasion of the oesophagus was limited to a circumscribed area of the muscular wall and could be resected completely at surgery should these cases be classified as T3 or T4? Metastases to the ipsilateral mediastinal nodes and subcarinal nodes remained within the N2 category, and a new N3 category was added to accommodate metastases to the contralateral mediastinal nodes, contralateral hilum or ipsilateral and contralateral supraclavicular or scalene lymph nodes. Additional changes in the new classification involved the moving of T1 N1 M0 cases from stage I to stage II and the division of stage III into IIIA, to accommodate T3 and N2 cases and IIIB, to accommodate the T4 and N3 categories (note, although stage subsets were identified by the use of the lower case in the original article by Dr. Mountain, upper case was now used for the first time in both the UICC and American manuals). The survival of those clinical and pathological TNM subsets that fell within stages I to IIIA and stage IV were shown to differ but no statistical analysis was presented. However, a graph showed statistically significant differences in survival between stage groupings. Once again there was no validation of any of the individual descriptors **contained** in these recommendations.

The AJCC published its 4th edition of TNM in 1992.(12) There were no changes for lung cancer. However, for the first time pleural mesothelioma was included, as a separate chapter.

At the time of the next revision in 1997 the database of Dr. Mountain had grown to include 5,319 cases, all but 66 being NSCLC. Of these, 4,351 cases had been treated at the M D Anderson Cancer Centre between 1975 and 1988 and documentation on a further 968 cases had been sent there from the National Cancer Institute cooperative Lung Cancer Study Group for confirmation of stage and histology. (13) Tables showed statistically significant differences in survival to 5 years between clinical/evaluative cTNM subsets and pathological/post-surgical pTNM subsets T1 N0 M0 and T2 N0 M0 and these were divided into a new stage IA and stage IB respectively. Similarly T1 N1 M0 cases were placed in a new stage IIA and T2 N1 M0 and T3 N0 M0 cases became stage IIB. The remaining TNM subsets in stages IIIA, IIIB and IV remained unchanged although statistically significant differences were found between some of these subsets. An additional paragraph determined that "the presence of *satellite* tumors within the primary-tumor lobe of the lung should be classified as T4. Intrapulmonary ispilateral *metastasis* in a distant, that is, nonprimary lobe(s) of the lung, should be classified M1." No data was presented to support these suggestions and the wording used to describe such additional pulmonary nodules was loaded to underline the apparent logic of considering some to be "satellite" lesions and therefore fell into a T category while those in other lobes were a "metastasis" and therefore fell into an M category. These recommendations were accepted by the AJCC and the UICC-TNM Prognostic Factors Project Committee, and were incorporated in to their 5th editions, published 1997. (14,15)

The International Association for the Study of Lung Cancer (IASLC) Lung Cancer Staging Project.

At an IASLC sponsored workshop in London in 1996 (16) Dr. Mountain presented his proposals for the forthcoming 5th edition of TNM. The Mountain database by this time had enlarged to include 5,319 cases, still relatively small, but this had been accumulated over 20 years, during which time many advances had been made in clinical staging, most importantly the routine application of computed tomography (CT) scanning. This database was mostly populated with surgical cases leading many oncologists unsure as to whether TNM had any relevance in non-surgical cases. The database reflected practice in one part of the world but informed an International classification. The lack of validation in previous editions of the TNM classification led to many of the descriptors being increasingly challenged by data from other sources. Because of these limitations, the delegates at the workshop felt that there was a need to develop a new database to inform future revisions of the TNM classification. It was suggested that the IASLC, as the only global organization dedicated to the study of lung cancer, representing all clinical and research aspects of lung cancer care, had a responsibility to become involved in the revision process. A proposal to this effect was included in the conclusions of the workshop (16) and placed before the board of the IASLC at the 8th World Conference on Lung Cancer held in Dublin in 1997. In December 1998 the board agreed to this proposal and granted pump-priming funds for the project. Meetings were held in London in 1999 and 2000 during which the composition of the committee was developed to ensure speciality and geographical representation and the involvement of stakeholders such as the UICC, the AJCC, the European Lung Cancer Working Group and the joint Japanese lung cancer societies. At the 9th World Conference held in Tokyo in 2000 the committee was joined by colleagues from Cancer Research And Biostatistics (CRAB), a not-for-profit medical statistics and data management organization based in Seattle with extensive experience with multi-centre data collection and analysis. At that meeting sufficient funds were guaranteed from the pharmaceutical industry to allow a major meeting in London in 2001 to which database proprietors were invited to present their data. Over the 2-day workshop data on 80,000 cases was presented from 20 databases across the globe. In was decided to base the budget required to continue this project upon the assumption that 30,000 suitable cases could be recruited and that the length of the project would be the 5-year cycle of revision proposed by the UICC and AJCC at that time. Cases would be solicited from databases world wide, treated by all modalities of care, registered between 1990 and 2000, a period during which there had been relative stability in staging methods. This would ensure a 5-year follow-up by the time of analysis. In collaboration with CRAB the data fields and data dictionary were finalized. Later that year full funding was obtained by the IASLC via a partnership agreement with a pharmaceutical company.

As the UICC and AJCC were aware of the progress of this initiative they decided that no changes should be made to lung cancer classification in the 6th editions of their manuals published in 2002. (17,18)

Meetings of the IASLC staging committee were held on an annual basis utilizing the World Conferences, now held biennially, wherever possible. In May 2003 the UICC and AJCC extended the revision cycle to 7 years and proposed that the 7th edition of the TNM would be published early in 2009. The internal review processes within these two organizations would require that the IASLC proposals be submitted to the UICC in January 2007 and the

AJCC in June 2008.

Data collection was discontinued in April 2005 by which time over 100,000 cases had been submitted to the data centre at CRAB. After an initial sift which excluded cases with insufficient data on stage, treatment or follow-up, cases outside the designated study period and cases in which the cell type was unsuited or unknown 81,495 were available for analysis, 68,463 cases

Table 1.1 Summary of cases contributed to the IASLC Staging Project.

Total Cases Submitted	100,869
Excluded From Current Analyses	19,374
- Outside of 1990-2000 Time Frame	5,467
- Incomplete Survival Data	1,192
- Unknown Histology	2,419
- Incomplete Stage Information	8,075
- Recurrent Cases and Other (e.g. Not known if recurrent vs. newly diagnosed, occult tumors)	1093
- Carcinoids, Sarcomas, other histologies	1,128
Included in Analyses	81,495
- SCLC	13,032
- NSCLC	68,463

of NSCLC and 13,032 cases of small-cell lung cancer (SCLC) (Table 1.1). The geographical distribution of the data sources is illustrated in Figure 1.3 and the spread of treatment modalities is shown in Figure 1.4.

At the 11th World Conference in Barcelona in June 2005 subcommittees were established to develop the proposals for key aspects of the proj-

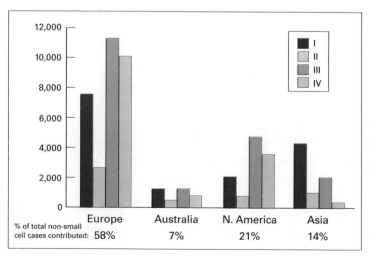

Figure 1.3 Geographical origin of data for IASLC Staging Project.

ect. Additional sub-groups were later added (Table 1.2). It was agreed that the membership of the IASLC, and the wider lung cancer community would be informed of the progress of the work through discussion articles to be published in the *Journal of Thoracic Oncology* (JTO), the official journal of the IASLC. (19)

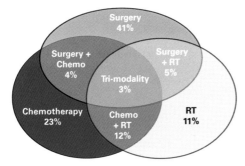

Figure 1.4 Treatment modalities of cases within the IASLC Staging Project.

Intensive validation was crucially important in this project and the lack of it in earlier editions had been a major motive for the development of the project. A validation and methodology subcommittee was therefore established and was intimately involved in the analyses conducted by CRAB and the development of the proposals from each sub-committee. (20) Internal validity was undertaken by ensuring that all of the proposals were supported across different types of databases and in most geographical areas. External validity was assured by testing the new proposals against the SEER data base for the relevant period.

Where the analyses showed descriptors to have a prognosis that differed from the other descriptors in any T or M category,

Table 1.2 Membership of the sub-committees of the IASLC Staging Project.

T-Descriptors
Chairperson Ramon Rami-Porta
David Ball
John Crowley
Peter Goldstraw
James Jett
William Travis
Masahiro Tsuboi
Eric Vallieres

N-Descriptors
Chairperson Valerie Rusch
John Crowley
Jung-Gi Im
Peter Goldstraw
Ryosuke Tsuchiya
Johan Vansteenkiste

Prognostic Factors
Chairperson Jean-Paul Sculier
John Crowley
Peter Goldstraw
Thierry Le Chevalier
Jan van Meerbeeck

Small Cell Lung Cancer
Chairperson Frances A. Shepherd
Desmond Carney
John Crowley
Peter Goldstraw
Paul Van Houtte
Pieter E. Postmus

Validation and Methodology
Chairperson Patti Groome
John Crowley
Peter Goldstraw
Catherine Kennedy
Leslie Sobin
Mark Krasnik

M-Descriptors
Chairperson Pieter Postmus
Elizabeth Brambilla
John Crowley
Peter Goldstraw
Ned Patz
Hiroyasu Yokomise

Nodal Chart
Chairperson: Ryosuke Tsuchiya
David Ball
John Crowley
Peter Goldstraw
Edward Patz

two alternative strategies were considered. First, retain that descriptor in the existing category, identified by alphabetical subscripts. For example, additional pulmonary nodules in the lobe of the primary, considered to be T4 in the 6th edition of TNM, would become T4a, while additional pulmonary nodules in other ipsilateral lobes, designated as M1 in the 6th edition, would become M1a. Second, allow descriptors to move between categories, to a category containing other descriptors with a similar prognosis, e.g. additional pulmonary nodules in the lobe of the primary would move from T4 to T3, and additional pulmonary nodules in other ipsilateral lobes would move from M1 to T4. The first strategy had the advantage of allowing, to a large extent, retrograde compatibility with existing databases. Unfortunately this generated a large number of descriptors (approximately 20) and an impractically large number of TNM subsets (over 180). For this reason backwards compatibility was compromised and strategy ii) was preferred for its clinical use. The resultant T, N, and M categories were incorporated into new TNM subsets and a small number of candidate stage groupings were developed using a recursive partitioning and amalgamation (RPA) algorithm. (21) The analysis grouped cases based on best stage (pathologic if available, otherwise clinical) after determination of best-split points based on overall survival on indicator variables for the newly proposed T/M categories and an ordered variable for N-category, excluding NX cases. This analysis was performed on a randomly selected training set comprising two-thirds of the available data that met the requirements for conversion to newly proposed T and M categories (N=17,726), reserving 9,133 cases for later validation. The random selection process was stratified by type of database submission and time period of case entry (1990-1995 vs 1995-2000). The RPA analysis generated a tree-based model for the survival data using log-rank test statistics for recursive partitioning and, for selection of the important groupings, bootstrap re-sampling to correct for the adaptive nature of the splitting algorithm. With an ordered list of groupings from the terminal nodes of the "survival tree" as a guide, several proposed stage groupings were created by combining adjacent groups. Selection of a final stage grouping proposal from among the candidate schemes was based upon its statistical properties in the training set and its relevance to clinical practice, and was arrived at by consensus.

The proposals from the project were submitted to the board of the IASLC in September 2006 and were approved unanimously. The recommendations regarding T, N, and M descriptors and the TNM stage groupings (22-25) were submitted to the UICC in December 2006 and to the AJCC in June 2007. The committee subsequently produced additional proposals: a) confirming and reinforcing the validity of the TNM classification in the clinical staging of SCLC, (26) b) demonstrating the use of TNM for the classification of broncho-pulmonary carcinoid tumors, (27) leading to the inclusion of carcinoid tumors for the first time in the 7th edition of TNM, c) the value of additional, and independent prognostic factors in the clinical and pathological TNM populations, (28,29) d) proposals for an international "IASLC" nodal chart that for the first time reconciled the differences in the Naruke and Mountain/Dresler nodal charts, allowing one chart to be used globally with consequent improvement in data collection and analysis, (30) and e) providing a clear definition of "visceral pleural invasion" a T2a descriptor. (31)

The IASLC Lung Cancer Staging Project has involved a great deal of work, not only from the members of the committee and our colleagues at CRAB but also from those Institutions that generously donated their data so that the project could succeed. The Lung Cancer community has much for which to thank these individuals.

The 7th edition of TNM in lung cancer is unique. It is the first classification to be based upon global data, data on cases treated by all modalities of care, and to have been intensively validated internally and externally. There will be questions raised about existing treatment algorithms. (32) It may be possible to get some data from the re-analysis of published studies but undoubtedly there will be a need for new prospective trials. The limitations inherent in a study that has been based upon retrospective data, notably imbalances and deficiencies in geographical recruitment and the spread of treatment modalities, and others, will be addressed in the next phase of the IASLC Staging Project. The prospective data set has been published(33) and a web-based data collection system is being developed. The project will be expanded to cover the neuroendocrine tumors of the lung, first covered by the WHO classification in 1999, (34,35) and mesothelioma. We hope that colleagues around the world will continue to support and contribute to this initiative, to ensure that the TNM classification is further improved in future editions.

References:

(1) Sellers TA. The Classification of Malignant Tumours by Anatomical Extent of Disease: The Development of the TNM System. 1980.

(2) Denoix PF. The TNM Staging System. *Bull Inst Nat Hyg* (Paris) 7, 743. 1952.

(3) UICC. TNM Classification of Malignant Tumours. 1st. 1968. Geneva, UICC.

(4) Mountain CF, Carr DT, Anderson WAD. A system for the clinical staging of lung cancer. Am J Roentgenol *Rad Ther Nucl Med* 120, 130-138. 1974.

(5) UICC. TNM Classification of Malignant Tumours. 2nd. 1975. Geneva, UICC.

(6) American Joint Committee on Cancer Staging and End Results Reporting. AJC Cancer Staging Manual. 1st ed. Philadelphia: Lippincott-Raven; 1977.

(7) UICC. TNM Classification of Malignant Tumours. 3rd. 1978. Geneva, UICC.

(8) American Joint Committee on Cancer. Manual for Staging of Cancer. Beahrs OH, Myers MH, editors. 2nd. 1983. Philadelphia, J.B. Lippincott Co.

(9) Mountain CF. A new international staging system for lung cancer. *Chest* 1986;89S:225S-32S.

(10) Hermanek P, Sobin LH, UICC. TNM Classification of Malignant Tumours. 4th. 1987. Berlin, Springer Verlag.

(11) American Joint Committee on Cancer. Manual for Staging of Cancer. Beahrs OH, Henson DE, Hutter RVP, Myers MH, editors. 3rd. 1988. Philadelphia, J.B. Lippincott Co.

(12) American Joint Committee on Cancer. Manual for Staging of Cancer. Beahrs OH, Henson DE, Hutter RVP, Kennedy BJ, editors. 4th. 1992. Philadelphia, J.B. Lippincott co.

(13) Mountain CF. Revisions in the International System for Staging Lung Cancer. Chest 111, 1710-1717. 1997.

(14) UICC International Union Against Cancer. TNM Classification of Malignant Tumours. Sobin LH, Wittekind C, editors. 5th. 1997. New York, Wiley-Liss.

(15) American Joint Committee on Cancer. AJCC Cancer Staging Manual. Fleming ID, Cooper JS, Henson DE, Hutter RVP, Kennedy BJ, Murphy GP et al., editors. 5th. 1997. Philadelphia, Lipincott Raven.

(16) Goldstraw P. Report on the International workshop on intrathoracic staging. London, October 1996. *Lung Cancer* 18, 107-111. 1997.

(17) UICC International Union Against Cancer. TNM Classification of Malignant Tumours. 6th ed. New York: Wiley-Liss; 2002.

(18) American Joint Committee on Cancer. AJCC Cancer Staging Manual. 6th ed. New York: Springer; 2002.

(19) Goldstraw P, Crowley J, IASLC International Staging Project. The IASLC International Staging Project on Lung Cancer. Journal of Thoracic Oncology 1, 281-286. 2006.

(20) Groome PA, Bolejack V, Crowley JJ, Kennedy C, Krasnik M, Sobin LH, et al. The IASLC Lung Cancer Staging Project: Validation of the proposals for revision of the T, N and M descriptors and consequent stage groupings in the forthcoming (seventh) TNM classification for lung cancer. *J Thorac Oncol* 2, 694-705. 2007.

(21) Crowley JJ, LeBlanc M, Jacobson J, et al. Some exploratory tools for survival analysis. In: Lin DY, Fleming TR, editors. Proceedings of the First Seattle Symposium in Biostatistics: Survival analysis.. 1st ed. New York: Springer; 1997. p. 199-229.

(22) Rami-Porta R, Ball D, Crowley JJ, Giroux DJ, Jett JR, Travis WD, et al. The IASLC Lung Cancer Staging Project: Proposals for the revision of the T descriptors in the forthcoming (seventh) edition of the TNM classification for lung cancer. *J Thorac Oncol* 2, 593-602. 2007.

(23) Rusch VR, Crowley JJ, Giroux DJ, Goldstraw P, Im J-G, Tsuboi M, et al. The IASLC Lung Cancer Staging Project: Proposals for revision of the N descriptors in the forthcoming (seventh) edition of the TNM classification for lung cancer. *J Thorac Oncol* 2, 603-612. 2007.

(24) Postmus PE, Brambilla E, Chansky K, Crowley J, Goldstraw P, Patz EF, et al. The IASLC Lung Cancer Staging Project: Proposals for revision of the M descriptors in the forthcoming (seventh) edition of the TNM classification for lung cancer. *J Thorac Oncol* 2, 686-693. 2007.

(25) Goldstraw P, Crowley JJ, Chansky K, Giroux DJ, Groome PA, Rami-Porta R, et al. The IASLC Lung Cancer Staging Project: Proposals for revision of the stage groupings in the forthcoming (seventh) edition of the TNM classification for lung cancer. *J Thorac Oncol* 2, 706-714. 2007.

(26) Shepherd FA, Crowley J, Van Houtte P, Postmus PE, Carney D, Chansky K, et al. The IASLC Lung Cancer Staging Project: Proposals regarding the clinical staging of small-cell lung cancer in the forthcoming (seventh) edition of the TNM classification for lung cancer. *J Thorac Oncol* 2, 1067-1077. 2007.

(27) Travis WD, Giroux DJ, Chansky K, Crowley J, Asamura H, Brambilla E, et al. The IASLC Lung Cancer Staging Project: Proposals for the inclusion of Bronchopulmonary Carcinoid tumours in the forthcoming (seventh) edition of the TNM Classification for Lung Cancer. *JThorac Oncol* 3, 1213-1223. 2008.

(28) Sculier JP, Chansky K, Crowley JJ, Van Meerbeeck J, Goldstraw P, IASLC International Staging Project. The impact of additional prognostic factors on survival and their relationship with the Anatomical Extent of Disease as expressed by the 6th edition of the TNM Classification of Malignant Tumours and the proposals for the 7th edition. *J Thorac Oncol* 3, 457-466. 2008.

(29) Chansky K, Sculier JP, Crowley JJ, Giroux DJ, Van Meerbeeck J, Goldstraw P, et al. The IASLC Lung Cancer Staging Project: Prognostic Factors and Pathologic TNM Stage in Surgically Managed Non-Small Cell Lung Cancer. *J Thorac Oncol* 4, 792-801. 2009.

(30) Rusch VW, Asamura H, Watanabe H, Giroux DJ, Rami-Porta R, Goldstraw P et al. The IASLC Lung Cancer Staging Project: A Proposal for a New International Lymph Node Map in the Forthcoming Seventh Edition of the TNM Classification for Lung Cancer. *J Thorac Oncol* 4, 568-577. 2009.

(31) Travis WD, Brambilla E, Rami-Porta R, Vallieres E, Tsuboi M, Rusch V, et al. Visceral pleural invasion: Pathologic criteria and use of elastic stains: Proposals for the 7th edition of the TNM Classification for Lung Cancer. *J Thorac Oncol* 3, 1384-1390. 2008.

(32) Goldstraw P. The 7th Edition of TNM for Lung Cancer: What now? *J Thorac Oncol* 4, 671-673. 2009.

(33) Giroux DJ, Rami-Porta R, Chansky K, Crowley JJ, Groome PA, Postmus PE, et al. The IASLC Lung Cancer Staging Project: Data Elements for the Prospective Project. *J Thorac Oncol* 4, 679-683. 2009.

(34) Travis WD, Brambilla E, Muller-Hermelink HK, Harris CC. World Health Organisation Classification of Tumours: Pathology and Genetics of Tumors of the Lung, Pleura, Thymus and Heart. Lyon: IARC Press; 2004.

(35) Lim E, Goldstraw P, Nicholson AG, Travis WD, Jett JR, Ferolla P, et al. Proceedings of the IASLC International Workshop on Advances in Neuroendocrine Tumors 2007. *J Thorac Oncol* 3, 1194-1201. 2008.

Editor's Note: The principles behind the TNM Classification of Malignant Tumours *have evolved over time and have become harmonized between the UICC and the AJCC. The general rules are important guidelines that not only establish immutable principles but also can assist the clinician in difficult cases where classification is in doubt. We reproduce here the latest version of the chapter from the UICC's TNM Classification of Malignant Tumours covering these principles. Further site-specific explanation of these general rules is given in Chapter 5: "Site-specific Explanatory Notes for Lung and Pleural Tumours" (page 64).*

Acknowledgment: Used with the permission of the International Union Against Cancer (UICC), Geneva, Switzerland. The original source for this material is the TNM Classification of Malignant Tumours 7th Edition *(2009) published by John Wiley & Sons Ltd, www.wiley.com.*

CHAPTER 2 | The Principles of the TNM System

The practice of dividing cancer cases into groups according to so-called stages arose from the fact that survival rates were higher for cases in which the disease was localized than for those in which the disease had extended beyond the organ of origin. These groups were often referred to as early cases and late cases, implying some regular progression with time. Actually, the stage of disease at the time of diagnosis may be a reflection not only of the rate of growth and extension of the neoplasm but also of the type of tumour and of the tumour-host relationship.

The staging of cancer is hallowed by tradition, and for the purpose of analysis of groups of patients it is often necessary to use such a method. The UICC believes that it is important to reach agreement on the recording of accurate information on the extent of the disease for each site, because the precise clinical description of malignant neoplasms and histopathological classification may serve a number of related objectives, namely

1. To aid the clinician in the planning of treatment
2. To give some indication of prognosis
3. To assist in evaluation of the results of treatment
4. To facilitate the exchange of information between treatment centres
5. To contribute to the continuing investigation of human cancer

The principal purpose to be served by international agreement on the classification of cancer cases by extent of disease is to provide a method of conveying clinical experience to others without ambiguity.

There are many bases or axes of tumour classification: for example, the anatomical site and the clinical and pathological extent of disease, the reported duration of symptoms or signs, the gender and age of the patient, and the histological type and grade. All of these bases or axes represent variables that are known to have an influence on the outcome of the disease. Classification by anatomical extent of disease as determined clinically and histopathologically (when possible) is the one with which the TNM system primarily deals.

The clinician's immediate task is to make a judgment as to prognosis and a decision as to the most effective course of treatment. This judgment and this decision require, among other things, an objective assessment of the anatomical extent of the disease. In accomplishing this, the trend is away from "staging" to meaningful description, with or without some form of summarization.

To meet the stated objectives a system of classification is needed
1. whose basic principles are applicable to all sites regardless of treatment; and
2. which may be supplemented later by information that becomes available from histopathology and/or surgery.

The TNM system meets these requirements.

The General Rules of the TNM System
The TNM system for describing the anatomical extent of disease is based on the assessment of three components:

T – The extent of the primary tumour
N – The absence or presence and extent of regional lymph node metastasis
M – The absence or presence of distant metastasis.

The addition of numbers to these three components indicates the extent of the malignant disease, thus:

T0, T1, T2, T3, T4 N0, N1, N2, N3 M0, M1

In effect the system is a "shorthand notation" for describing the extent of a particular malignant tumour.

The general rules applicable to all sites are as follows:
1. All cases should be confirmed microscopically. Any cases not so proved must be reported separately.
2. Two classifications are described for each site, namely:

(a) Clinical classification (Pre-treatment clinical classification), designated TNM (or cTNM) is essential to select and evaluate therapy. This is based on evidence acquired before treatment. Such evidence arises from physical examination, imaging, endoscopy, biopsy, surgical exploration, and other relevant examinations.

(b) Pathological classification (Post-surgical histopathological classification), designated pTNM provides the most precise data to estimate prognosis and calculate end results. This is based on the evidence acquired before treatment, supplemented or modified by the additional evidence acquired from surgery and from pathological examination. The pathological assessment of the primary tumour (pT) entails a resection of the primary tumour or biopsy adequate to evaluate the highest pT category. The pathological assessment of the regional lymph nodes (pN) entails removal of nodes adequate to validate the absence of regional lymph node metastasis (pN0). An excisional biopsy alone of a lymph node without pathological assessment of the primary is insufficient to fully evaluate the pN category and is a clinical classification, the exception being a biopsy of a sentinel node. The pathological assessment of distant metastasis (pM) entails microscopic examination.

3. After assigning T, N, and M and/or pT, pN, and pM categories, these may be grouped into stages. The TNM classification and stage grouping, once established, must remain unchanged in the medical records.

4. If there is doubt concerning the correct T, N, or M category to which a particular case should be allotted, then the lower (i.e., less advanced) category should be chosen. This will also be reflected in the stage grouping.

5. In the case of multiple simultaneous tumours in one organ, the tumour with the highest T category should be classified and the multiplicity or the number of tumours should be indicated in parentheses, e.g., T2 (m) or T2 (5). In simultaneous bilateral cancers of paired organs, each tumour should be classified independently. In tumours of the liver, ovary, and fallopian tube, multiplicity is a criterion of T classification.

6. Definitions of TNM categories and stage grouping may be telescoped or expanded for clinical or research purposes as long as basic definitions recommended are not changed. For instance, any T, N, or M can be divided into subgroups.

Anatomical Regions and Sites

The sites in this classification are listed by code number of the International Classification of Diseases for Oncology (1). Each region or site is described

under the following headings:
- Rules for classification with the procedures for assessing the T, N, and M categories
- Anatomical sites, and subsites if appropriate
- Definition of the regional lymph nodes
- TNM Clinical classification
- pTNM Pathological classification
- G Histopathological grading
- Stage grouping
- Summary for the region or site

TNM Clinical Classification

The following general definitions are used throughout:

T – Primary Tumour

TX   Primary tumour cannot be assessed

T0   No evidence of primary tumour

Tis   Carcinoma in situ

T1, T2, T3, T4 Increasing size and/or local extent of the primary tumour

N – Regional Lymph Nodes

NX   Regional lymph nodes cannot be assessed

N0   No regional lymph node metastasis

N1, N2, N3 Increasing involvement of regional lymph nodes

Notes: Direct extension of the primary tumour into lymph nodes is classified as lymph node metastasis. Metastasis in any lymph node other than regional is classified as a distant metastasis.

M – Distant Metastasis*

M0   No distant metastasis

M1   Distant metastasis

The MX category is considered to be inappropriate as clinical assessment of metastasis can be based on physical examination alone. (The use of MX may result in exclusion from cancer registration).

The category M1 may be further specified according to the following notation:

Pulmonary	PUL (C34)	Bone marrow	MAR (C42.1)
Osseous	OSS (C40,41)	Pleura	PLE (C38.4)
Hepatic	HEP (C22)	Peritoneum	PER (C48.1,2)
Brain	BRA (C71)	Adrenals	ADR (C74)

Lymph nodes LYM (C77)   Skin   SKI   (C44)
Others   OTH

Subdivisions of TNM
Subdivisions of some main categories are available for those who need greater specificity (e.g., Tla, lb or N2a, 2b).

pTNM Pathological Classification
The following general definitions are used throughout:
pT – Primary Tumour
pTX   Primary tumour cannot be assessed histologically
pT0   No histological evidence of primary tumour
pTis   Carcinoma in situ
pTl, pT2, pT3, pT4 Increasing size and/or local extent of the primary
        tumour histologically

pN – Regional Lymph Nodes
pNX   Regional lymph nodes cannot be assessed histologically
pN0   No regional lymph node metastasis histologically
pN1, pN2, pN3 Increasing involvement of regional lymph nodes histo-
        logically

Notes: 1. Direct extension of the primary tumour into lymph nodes is classified as lymph node metastasis.
2. Tumour deposits (satellites), i.e., macro- or microscopic nests or nodules, in the lymph drainage area of a primary carcinoma without histologic evidence of residual lymph node in the nodule, may represent discontinuous spread, venous invasion with extravascular spread (V1/2) or a totally replaced lymph node. If a nodule is considered by the pathologist to be a totally replaced lymph node (generally having a smooth contour), it should be recorded as a positive lymph node, and each such nodule should be counted separately as a lymph node in the final pN determination.
3. When size is a criterion for pN classification, measurement is made of the metastasis, not of the entire lymph node.
4. Cases with micrometastasis only, i.e., no metastasis larger than 0.2 cm, can be identified by the addition of "(mi)", e.g., pNl(mi) or pN2(mi)

Sentinel Lymph Node
The sentinel lymph node is the first lymph node to receive lymphatic drainage from a primary tumour. If it contains metastatic tumour this indicates

that other lymph nodes may contain tumour. If it does not contain metastatic tumour, other lymph nodes are not likely to contain tumour. Occasionally there is more than one sentinel lymph node.

The following designations are applicable when sentinel lymph node assessment is attempted:

pNX(sn)   Sentinel lymph node could not be assessed

pN0(sn)   No sentinel lymph node metastasis

pNl-3 (sn) Sentinel lymph node metastasis

Isolated Tumour Cells

Isolated tumour cells (ITC) are single tumour cells or small clusters of cells not more than 0.2 mm in greatest dimension that are detected by routine (H&E) stains or immunohistochemistry. ITCs do not typically show evidence of metastatic activity (e.g., proliferation or stromal reaction) or penetration of vascular or lymphatic sinus walls. Cases with ITC in lymph nodes or at distant sites should be classified as N0 or M0, respectively. The same applies to cases with findings suggestive of tumour cells or their components by non-morphologic techniques such as flow cytometry or DNA analysis. These cases should be analysed separately. The classification is as follows (2).

N0   No regional lymph node metastasis histologically, no
           examination for isolated tumour cells(ITC)

pN0(i–)   No regional lymph node metastasis histologically, negative
           morphological findings for ITC

pN0(i+)   No regional lymph node metastasis histologically, positive
           morphological findings for ITC

pN0(mol–) No regional lymph node metastasis histologically, negative
           non-morphological findings for ITC

pN0(mol+) No regional lymph node metastasis histologically, positive
           non-morphological findings for ITC

Cases with or examined for isolated tumour cells (ITC) in sentinel lymph nodes can be classified in a similar manner. For example:

pN0(i+)(sn) No sentinel lymph node metastasis histologically, positive
             morphological findings for ITC

pM – Distant Metastasis*
   pM0 No distant metastasis microscopically
   pM1 Distant metastasis microscopically
   pMX is not a valid category

The category pMl may be further specified in the same way as M1 (see pages 34-35).

Isolated tumour cells found in bone marrow with morphological techniques are classified according to the scheme for N, e.g., M0(i+). For non-morphologic findings "mol" is used in addition to M0, e.g., M0(mol+).

Subdivisions of pTNM
Subdivisions of some main categories are available for those who need greater specificity (e.g., pT1a, lb or pN2a, 2b).

Histopathological Grading
In most sites further information regarding the primary tumour may be recorded under the following heading:
G – Histopathological Grading
GX   Grade of differentiation cannot be assessed
G1   Well differentiated
G2   Moderately differentiated
G3   Poorly differentiated
G4   Undifferentiated

Notes: Grades 3 and 4 can be combined in some circumstances as "G3-4, Poorly differentiated or undifferentiated." The bone and soft tissue sarcoma classifications also use "high grade" and "low grade."

Additional Descriptors
For identification of special cases in the TNM or pTNM classification, the "m", "y", "r", and "a" symbols are used. Although they do not affect the stage grouping, they indicate cases needing separate analysis.
m Symbol. The suffix m, in parentheses, is used to indicate the presence of multiple primary tumours at a single site. See TNM rule no. 5 (see page 33).
y Symbol. In those cases in which classification is performed during or following initial multimodality therapy, the cTNM or pTNM category is identified by a y prefix. The ycTNM or ypTNM categorizes the extent of tumour actually present at the time of that examination. The y categorization is not

an estimate of the extent of tumour prior to multimodality therapy.

r Symbol. Recurrent tumours, when classified after a disease-tree interval, are identified by the prefix r.

a Symbol. The prefix a indicates that classification is first determined at autopsy.

Optional Descriptors

L – Lymphatic Invasion
LX   Lymphatic invasion cannot be assessed
L0   No lymphatic invasion
L I   Lymphatic invasion

V – Venous Invasion
VX   Venous invasion cannot be assessed
V0   No venous invasion
VI   Microscopic venous invasion
V2   Macroscopic venous invasion

Note: Macroscopic involvement of the wall of veins (with no tumour within the veins) is classified as V2.

C-Factor

The C-factor, or certainty factor, reflects the validity of classification according to the diagnostic methods employed. Its use is optional.

The C-factor definitions are:

C1 Evidence from standard diagnostic means (e.g., inspection, palpation, and standard radiography, intraluminal endoscopy for tumours of certain organs)

C2 Evidence obtained by special diagnostic means (e.g., radiographic imaging in special projections, tomography, computerized tomography [CT], ultrasonography, lymphography, angiography; scintigraphy; magnetic resonance imaging [MRI]; endoscopy, biopsy, and cytology)

C3 Evidence from surgical exploration, including biopsy and cytology

C4 Evidence of the extent of disease following definitive surgery and pathological examination of the resected specimen

C5 Evidence from autopsy

Example: Degrees of C may be applied to the T, N, and M categories. A case might be described as T3C2, N2C1, M0C2.

The TNM clinical classification is therefore equivalent to C1, C2, and C3 in varying degrees of certainty, while the pTNM pathological classification generally is equivalent to C4.

Residual Tumour (R) Classification

The absence or presence of residual tumour after treatment is described by the symbol R.

TNM and pTNM describe the anatomical extent of cancer in general without considering treatment. They can be supplemented by the R classification, which deals with tumour status after treatment. It reflects the effects of therapy, influences further therapeutic procedures and is a strong predictor of prognosis.

The definitions of the R categories are:

RX   Presence of residual tumour cannot be assessed

R0   No residual tumour

R1   Microscopic residual tumour

R2   Macroscopic residual tumour

Some consider the R Classification to apply only to the primary tumour and its local or regional extent. Others have applied it more broadly to include distant metastasis. The specific usage chosen should be indicated when the R is used.

Stage Grouping

Classification by the TNM system achieves reasonably precise description and recording of the apparent anatomical extent of disease. A tumour with four degrees of T, three degrees of N, and two degrees of M will have 24 TNM categories. For purposes of tabulation and analysis, except in very large series, it is necessary to condense these categories into a convenient number of TNM stage groups.

Carcinoma in situ is categorized stage 0; cases with distant metastasis stage IV (except at certain sites, e.g., papillary and follicular carcinoma of thyroid).

The grouping adopted is such as to ensure, as far as possible, that each group is more or less homogeneous in respect of survival, and that the survival rates of these groups for each cancer site are distinctive.

For pathological stage grouping, if sufficient tissue has been removed for pathologic examination to evaluate the highest T and N categories, M1 may be either clinical (cM 1) or pathologic (pM1). However, if only a distant metastasis has had microscopic confirmation, the classification is pathologic (pM1) and the stage is pathologic.

Anatomical extent of disease as categorized by TNM is the most powerful prognostic indicator for the vast majority of malignancies; however it has been recognized for some time that factors other than anatomical extent of disease have a significant impact on predicting survival at diagnosis. This has resulted in the incorporation of some of these factors into stage grouping, e.g., age in thyroid cancer, and grade in soft tissue sarcoma. As more prognostic factors become available and their significance validated, an effort will be made to incorporate them along with anatomic factors to produce prognostic groups.

References:

(1) Fritz A, Percy C, Jack A, Shanmugaratnam K, Sobin L, Parkin DM, Whelan S, eds. *WHO International Classification of Diseases for Oncology ICD-O*, 3rd ed. Geneva: WHO; 2000.

(2) Hermanek P, Hutter RVP, Sobin LH, Wittekind Ch. Classification of isolated tumor cells and micrometastasis. *Cancer* 1999;86:2668-2673.

Editor's Note: One of the purposes of the TNM classification is "to give some indication of prognosis." This chapter, contributed by the AJCC, provides an overview of the statistical principles and methodologies used to assess prognosis. The strengths and pitfalls inherent in each analytical method are highlighted to show the importance of choosing the correct statistical tool in each situation.

Acknowledgment: Used with the permission of the American Joint Committee on Cancer. The original source of this material is the AJCC Cancer Staging Handbook (6th edition; 2002, © American Joint Committee on Cancer, Springer Science + Business Media, LLC). Published by Springer Science + Business Media, LLC, www.springer.com.

CHAPTER 3 | Cancer Survival Analysis

Analysis of cancer survival data and related outcomes are quantitative tools commonly used to access cancer treatment programs and to monitor the progress of regional and national cancer control programs. In this chapter the most common survival analysis methodology will be illustrated, basic terminology will be defined, and the essential elements of data collection and reporting will be described. Although the underlying principles are applicable to both, the focus of this discussion will be on the use of survival analysis to describe data typically available in cancer registries rather than to analyze research data obtained from clinical trials or laboratory experimentation. Discussion of statistical principles and methodology will be limited. Persons interested in statistical underpinnings or research applications are referred to textbooks that explore these topics at length (Cox and Oakes, 1984; Fleming and Harrington, 1991; Kalbfleisch and Prentice, 1980; Kleinbaum, 1996; Lee, 1992).

Basic Concepts

A *survival rate* is a statistical index that summarizes the probable frequency of specific outcomes for a group of patients at a particular point in time. A *survival curve* is a summary display of the pattern of survival rates over time. The basic concept is simple. For example, for a certain category of patient, one might ask what proportion are likely to be alive at the end of a specified interval, such as 5 years. The greater the proportion surviving, the more effective the program. Survival analysis, however, is somewhat more complicated than it first might appear. If one were to measure the length of time between diagnosis and death or record the vital status when last observed for every patient in a selected patient group, one might be tempted to describe the survival of a group as the proportion alive at the end of the period under investigation. This simple measure will be informative, however, only if all of the patients were observed for the same length of time.

In most real situations, it is not the case that all members of the group are observed for the same amount of time. Patients diagnosed near the end of the study period are more likely to be alive at last contact and will have been followed for less time than those diagnosed earlier. Even though it was not possible to follow these persons as long as the others, their survival might eventually have proved to be just as long or longer. Another difficulty is that it usually is not possible to know the outcome status of all of the persons who were in the group at the beginning. People move or change names and are lost to follow-up. Some of these persons may have died and others could be still living. Thus, if a survival rate is to describe the outcomes for an entire group accurately, there must be some means to deal with the fact that different persons in the group are observed for different lengths of time and that for others, their vital status is not known at the time of analysis. In the language of survival analysis, subjects who are observed until they reach the endpoint of interest (e.g., death) are called *uncensored* cases, and those who survive beyond the end of the follow-up or who are lost to follow-up at some point are termed *censored* cases.

Two basic survival procedures that enable one to determine overall group survival, taking into account both censored and uncensored observations, are the life table method (Berkson and Gage, 1950) and the Kaplan-Meier method (Kaplan-Meier, 1958). The life table method was the first method generally used to describe cancer survival results, and it came to be known as the actuarial method because of its similarity to the work done by actuaries in the insurance industry. The specific method of computation, i.e., life table or Kaplan-Meier, should always be indicated to avoid any confusion associated with the use of less precise terminology. Rates computed by different methods are not directly comparable, and when the survival experiences of different patient groups are compared, the different rates must be computed by the same method.

The illustrations in this chapter are based on data obtained from public-use files of the National Cancer Institute Surveillance, Epidemiology, and End Results (SEER) program. The cases selected are a 1% random sample of the total number for selected sites and years of diagnosis. Follow-up of these patients continued through the end of 1999. Thus, for the earliest patients, there can be as much as 16 years of follow-up, but for those diagnosed at the end of the study period, there can be as little as 1 year of follow-up. These data are used both because they are realistic in terms of the actual survival rates they yield and because they encompass a number of cases that might be seen in a single large tumor registry over a comparable number of years. They are intended only to illustrate the methodology. SEER results from 1973 to 1997 are more fully described elsewhere (Ries et al., 2000) and these illustrations should not be regarded as an adequate description of the total or current United States patterns of breast or lung cancer survival.

The Life Table Method

The life table method involves dividing the total period over which a group is observed into fixed intervals, usually months or years. For each interval, the proportion surviving to the end of the interval is calculated on the basis of the number known to have experienced the endpoint event (e.g., death) during the interval and the number estimated to have been at risk at the start of the interval. For each succeeding interval, a cumulative survival rate may be calculated. The cumulative survival rate is the probability of surviving the most recent interval multiplied by the probabilities of surviving all of the prior intervals. Thus, if the percent of the patients surviving the first interval is 90% and is the same for the second and third intervals, the cumulative survival percentage is 72.9% (.9 x .9 x .9 = .729).

Results from the life table method for calculating survival for the breast cancer illustration are shown in Figure 3.1. Two thousand eight hundred nineteen (2,819) patients diagnosed between 1983 and 1998 were followed through 1999. Following the life table calculation method for each year after diagnosis, the 1-year survival rate is 95.6%. The 5-year cumulative survival rate is 76.8%. At 10 years, the cumulative survival is 61.0%.

The lung cancer data show a much different survival pattern (Fig. 3.2). At 1 year following diagnosis, the survival rate is only 41.8%. By 5 years it has fallen to 12.0% and only 6.8% of lung cancer patients are estimated to have survived for 10 years following diagnosis. For lung cancer patients the *median survival time* is 10.0 months. Median survival time is the amount of time required to pass so that half the patients have experienced the end point event and half the patients remain event-free. If the cumulative survival does not fall below 50% it is not possible to estimate median survival from the data, as is the case in the breast cancer data.

In the case of breast cancer, the 10-year survival rate is important because such a large proportion of patients live more than 5 years past their

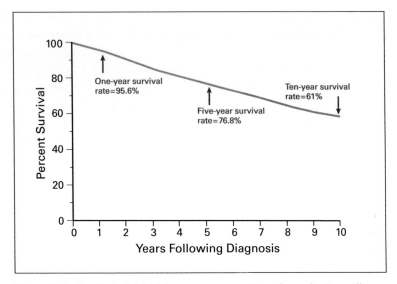

Figure 3.1 Survival of 2,819 breast cancer patients from the Surveillance, Epidemiology, and End Results Program of the National Cancer Institute, 1983-1998. Calculated by the life table method.

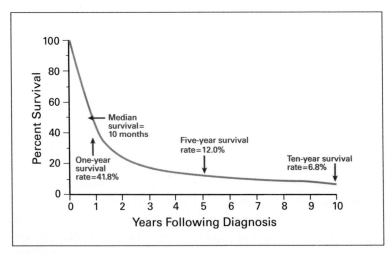

Figure 3.2 Survival of 2,347 lung cancer patients from the Surveillance, Epidemiology, and End Results Program of the National Cancer Institute, 1983-1998. Calculated by the life table method.

diagnosis. The 10-year time frame for lung cancer is less meaningful because such a large proportion of this patient group dies well before that much time passes.

An important assumption of all actuarial survival methods is that censored cases do not differ from the entire collection of uncensored cases in any systematic manner that would affect their survival. For example, if the more recently diagnosed cases in Figure 3.1, i.e., those who were most likely not to have died yet tended to be detected with earlier-stage disease than the uncensored cases; or if they were treated differently the assumption about comparability of censored and uncensored cases would not be met, and the result for the group as a whole would be inaccurate. Thus it is important, when patients are included in a life table analysis, that one be reasonably confident that differences in the amount of information available about survival are not related to differences that might affect survival.

The Kaplan-Meier Method

These same data can be analyzed using the Kaplan-Meier method (Kaplan and Meier, 1958). It is similar to the life table method but provides for calculating the proportion surviving to each point in time that a death occurs, rather than at fixed intervals. The principal difference evident in a survival curve is that the stepwise changes in the cumulative survival rate appear to occur independently of the intervals on the Years Following Diagnosis axis.

Patient-, Disease-, and Treatment-Specific Survival

Although overall group survival is informative, comparisons of the overall survival between two groups often are confounded by differences in the patients, their tumors, or the treatments they received. For example, it would be misleading to compare the overall survival depicted in Figure 3.1 with the overall survival of other breast cancer patients who tend to be diagnosed with more advanced disease, whose survival would be presumed to be poorer. The simplest approach to accounting for possible differences between groups is to provide survival results that are specific to the categories of patient, disease, or treatment that may affect results. In most cancer applications the most important variable by which survival results should be subdivided is the stage of disease. Figure 3.3 shows the *stage-specific* 5-year survival curves of the same breast cancer patients described earlier. These data show that breast cancer patient survival differs markedly according to the stage of the tumor at the time of diagnosis.

Almost any variable can be used to subclassify survival rates, but some are more meaningful than others. For example, it would be pos-

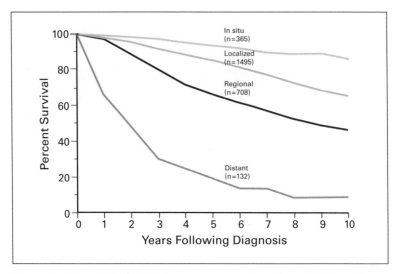

Figure 3.3 Survival of 2,819 breast cancer patients from the Surveillance, Epidemiology, and End Results Program of the National Cancer Institute, 1983-1998. Calculated by the life table method and stratified by historic stage of disease. Note: Excludes 119 patients with unknown state of disease. SEER uses extent of disease (EOD) staging.

sible to provide season-of-diagnosis-specific (i.e., spring, summer, winter, fall) survival rates, but the season of diagnosis probably has no biologic association with the length of a breast cancer patient's survival. On the other hand, the race-specific and age-specific survival rates shown in Figures 3.4 and 3.5 suggest that both of these variables are related to breast cancer survival. Whites have the highest survival rates and African-Americans the lowest. In the case of age, these data suggest that only the oldest patients experience poor survival and that it would be helpful to consider the effects of other causes of death that affect older persons using adjustments to be described.

Although the factors that affect survival may be unique to each type of cancer, it has become conventional that a basic description of survival for a specific cancer should include stage, age, and race-specific survival results. Treatment is a factor by which survival is commonly subdivided but it must be kept in mind that selection of treatment is usually related to some other factors which exert influence on survival. For example, in cancer care the choice of treatment is often dependent on the stage of disease at diagnosis.

Adjusted Survival Rate

The survival rates depicted in the illustrations account for all deaths, regardless of cause. This is known as *observed survival rate*. Although observed

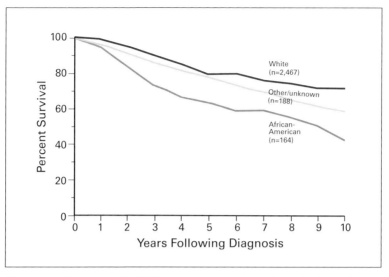

Figure 3.4 Survival of 2,819 breast cancer patients from the Surveillance, Epidemiology, and End Results Program of the National Cancer Institute, 1983-1998. Calculated by the life table method and stratified by race.

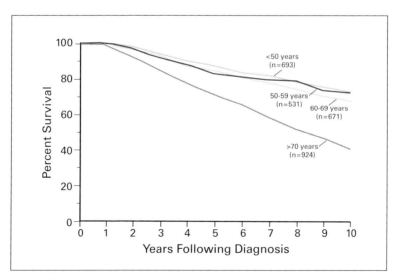

Figure 3.5 Survival of 2,819 breast cancer patients from the Surveillance, Epidemiology, and End Results Program of the National Cancer Institute, 1983-1998. Calculated by the life table method and stratified by age at diagnosis.

survival is a true reflection of total mortality in the patient group, we frequently are interested in describing mortality attributable only to the disease under investigation. The *adjusted survival rate* is the proportion of the initial patient group that escaped death due to a specific cause (e.g., cancer) if no other cause of death was operating. Whenever reliable information on cause of death is available, an adjustment can be made for deaths due to causes other than the disease under study. This is accomplished by treating patients who died without the disease of interest as censored observations. If adjusted survival rates were calculated for lung cancer, the pattern of survival would show little difference between observed and adjusted rates, because lung cancer usually is the cause of death for patients with the diagnosis. For diseases with more favorable survival patterns, such as breast cancer, patients live long enough to be at risk of other causes of death, and in these instances, adjusted survival rates will tend to be higher than observed survival rates and to give a clearer picture of the specific effects of the diagnosis under investigation. Adjusted rates can be calculated for either life table or Kaplan-Meier results.

Relative Survival

Information on cause of death is sometimes unavailable or unreliable. Under such circumstances, it is not possible to compute an adjusted survival rate. However, it is possible to adjust partially for differences in the risk of dying from causes other than the disease under study. This can be done by means of the *relative survival rate*, which is the ratio of the observed survival rate to the expected rate for a group of people in the general population similar to the patient group with respect to race, sex, and age. The relative survival rate is calculated using a procedure described by Ederer, Axtell, and Cutler (1961).

The relative survival rate represents the likelihood that a patient will not die from causes associated specifically with their cancer at some specified time after diagnosis. It is always larger than observed survival rate for the same group of patients. If the group is sufficiently large and the patients are roughly representative of the population of the United States (taking race, sex, and age into account), the relative survival rate provides a useful estimate of the probability of escaping death from the specific cancer under study. However, if reliable information on cause of death is available, it is preferable to use the adjusted rate. This is particularly true when the series is small or when the patients are largely drawn from a particular socioeconomic segment of the population. Relative survival rates may be derived from life table or Kaplan-Meier results.

Regression Methods

Examining survival within specific patient, disease, or treatment categories is the simplest way of studying multiple factors possibly associated with survival. This approach, however, is limited to factors into which patients may be broadly grouped. This approach does not lend itself to studying the effects of measures that vary on an interval scale. There are many examples of interval variables in cancer, such as number of positive nodes, cell counts, and laboratory marker values. If the patient population were to be divided up into each interval value, too few subjects would be in each analysis to be meaningful. In addition, when more than one factor is considered, the number of curves that result provide so many comparisons that the effects of the factors defy interpretation.

Conventional multiple regression analysis investigates the joint effects of multiple variables on a single outcome, but it is incapable of dealing with censored observations. For this reason, other statistical methods have had to be developed to assess the relationship of survival time to a number of variables simultaneously. The most commonly used is the Cox proportional hazards regression model (Cox, 1972). This model provides a method for estimating the influence of multiple covariates on the survival distribution from data that include censored observations. Covariates are the multiple factors to be studied in association with survival. In the Cox proportional hazards regression model, the covariates may be categorical variables such as race, interval measures such as age, or laboratory test results.

Specifics of these methods are beyond the scope of this chapter. Fortunately, many readily accessible computer packages for statistical analysis now permit the methods to be applied quite easily by the knowledgeable analyst. Although much useful information can be derived from multivariate survival models, they generally do require additional assumptions about the shape of the survival curve and the nature of the effects of covariates. One must always examine the appropriateness of the model that is used relative to the assumptions required.

Standard Error of a Survival Rate

Survival rates that describe the experience of the specific group of patients are frequently used to generalize to larger populations. The existence of true population values is postulated, and these values are estimated from the group under study, which is only a sample of the larger population. If a survival rate were calculated from a second sample taken from the same population, it is unlikely that the results would be exactly the same. The difference between the two results is called the sampling variation (chance variation or sampling error). The *standard error* is a measure of the extent to which sampling variation influences the computed survival rate. In repeated observations under the same conditions, the true or population survival rate will lie within the range of two standard errors on either side of the computed rate about 95 times in 100. This range is called the 95% *confidence interval*.

Comparison or Survival Between Patient Groups

In comparing survival rates of two patient groups, the statistical significance of the observed difference is of interest. The essential question is "What is the probability that the observed difference may have occurred by chance?" The standard error of the survival rate provides a simple means for answering this question. If the 95% confidence intervals of two survival rates do not overlap, the observed difference would customarily be considered statistically significant—that is, unlikely to be due to chance.

It is possible that the differences between two groups at each comparable time of follow-up do not differ significantly but that when the survival curves are considered in their entirely, the individual insignificant differences combine to yield a significantly different pattern of survival. The most common statistical test that examines the whole pattern of differences between survival curves is the *log rank test*. This test equally weights the effects of differences occurring throughout the follow-up and is the appropriate choice for most situations. Other tests weight the differences according to the numbers of persons at risk at different points and can yield different results depending on whether deaths tend more to occur early or later in the follow-up.

Care must be exercised in the interpretation of tests of statistical significance. For example, if differences exist in the patient and disease characteristics of two treatment groups, a statistically significant difference in survival results may primarily reflect differences between the two patient series, rather than differences inefficacy of the treatment regimens. The more definitive approach to therapy evaluation requires a randomized clinical trial that helps to ensure comparability of the patient characteristics and the disease characteristics of the two treatment groups.

Definition of Study Starting Point

The starting time for determining survival of patients depends on the purpose of the study. For example, the starting time for studying the natural history of a particular cancer might be defined in reference t the appearance of the first symptom. Various reference dates are commonly used as starting times for evaluating the effects of therapy. These include (1) date of diagnosis, (2) date of the first visit to physician or clinic, (3) date of hospital admission, and (4) date of treatment initiation. If the time to recurrence of a tumor after apparent complete remission is being studied, the starting time is the date of apparent complete remission. The specific reference date used should be clearly specified in every report.

The date of initiation of therapy should be used as the starting time for evaluating therapy. For untreated patients, the most comparable date is the time at which it was decided that no tumor-directed treatment would be given. For both treated and untreated patients, the above times from which survival rates are calculated will usually coincide with the date of the initial staging of cancer.

Vital Status
At any given time, the vital status of each patient is defined as alive, dead, or unknown (i.e., lost to follow-up). The endpoint of each patient's participation in the study is (1) a specified "terminal event" such as death, (2) survival to the completion of the study, or (3) loss to follow-up. In each case, the observed follow-up time is the time from the starting point to the terminal event, to the end of the study, or to the date of last observation. This observed follow-up may be further described in terms of patient status at the endpoint, such as

Alive; tumor-free; no recurrence

Alive; tumor-free; after recurrence

Alive with persistent, recurrent, or metastatic disease

Alive with primary tumor

Dead; tumor free

Dead; with cancer (primary, recurrent, or metastatic disease)

Dead; postoperative

Unknown; lost to follow-up

Completeness of the follow-up is crucial in any study of survival, because even a small number of patients lost to follow-up may lead to inaccurate or biased results. The maximum possible effect of bias from patients lost to follow-up may be ascertained by calculating a maximum survival rate, assuming that all lost patients lived to the end of the study. A minimum survival rate may be calculated by assuming that all patients lost to follow-up died at the time they were lost.

Time Intervals
The total survival time is often divided into intervals in units of weeks, months, or years. The survival curve for these intervals provides a descrip-

tion of the population under study with respect to the dynamics of survival over a specified time. The time interval used should be selected with regard to the natural history of the disease under consideration. In diseases with a long natural history, the duration of study could be 5 to 20 years, and survival intervals of 6 to 12 months will provide a meaningful description of the survival dynamics. If the population being studied has a very poor prognosis (e.g., patients with carcinoma of the esophagus or pancreas), the total duration of study may be 2 to 3 years, and the survival intervals may be described in terms of 1 to 3 months. In interpreting survival rates, one must also take into account the number of individuals entering a survival interval.

Summary

This chapter has reviewed the rudiments of survival analysis as it is often applied to cancer registry data. Complex analysis of data and exploration of research hypotheses demand greater knowledge and expertise than could be conveyed herein. Survival analysis is now performed automatically in many different registry data management and statistical analysis programs available for use on personal computers. Persons with access to these programs are encouraged to explore the different analysis features available to demonstrate for themselves the insight on cancer registry data that survival analysis can provide.

Bibliography:

American Joint Committee on Cancer: AJCC Cancer Staging Manual, 5th ed. Fleming ID, Cooper JS, Henson DE et al (Eds.). Philadelphia: Lippincott-Raven, 1997

Berkson J, Gage RP: Calculation of survival rates for cancer. Proc Staff Meet Mayo Clinic 25:270-286, 1950

Cox DR: Regression models and life tables. J R Stat Soc B 34:187-220, 1972

Cox DR, Oakes D: Analysis of survival data. London: Chapman and Hall, 1984

Ederer F, Axtell LM, Cutler SJ: The relative survival rate: a statistical methodology. Natl Cancer Inst Monogr 6:101-121, 1961

Fleming TR, Harrington DP: Counting processes and survival analysis. New York: John Wiley, 1991

Kalbfleisch JD, Prentice RL: The statistical analysis of failure time data. New York: John Wiley, 321, 1980

Kaplan EL, Meier P: Nonparametric estimation from incomplete observations. J Am Stat Assn 53:457-481, 1958

Kleinbaurn DG: Survival analysis: a self learning text. New York: Springer-Verlag, 1996

Lee ET: Statistical methods for survival data analysis. New York: John Wiley, 1992

Mantel N: Evaluation of survival data and two new rank order statistics arising in its consideration. Cancer Chemother Rep 50:163-170, 1966

Ries LAG, Eisner MP, Kosary CL, et al (Eds.): SEER cancer statistics review, 1973-1997: tables and graphs, National Cancer Institute. Bethesda, MD: National Institutes of Health, NIH Pub. No.00-2789, 2000

Editor's Note: This, the seventh edition of the TNM Classification of Malignant Tumours, *represents the first revision of the* TNM *classification for lung cancer since the fifth edition in 1997; no changes being made to the sixth edition published in 2002. The revisions are entirely based on the recommendations of the IASLC Staging Project, derived from the IASLC International Database for Lung Cancer, and were accepted without change by the UICC and the AJCC. There are changes to some T and M categories and certain stage categories. However, the most important change is that within the process for change itself. Through its foresight in establishing its Staging Project, the IASLC, on behalf of its members and the thoracic oncology com¬munity, has earned a central role in future revisions and will ensure that these are relevant to patients being treated by all modalities of care around the world. This chapter is a summary of the new classification. Further information and site-specific explanations are given in later chapters.*

Acknowledgment: Used with the permission of the International Union Against Cancer (UICC), Geneva, Switzerland. The original source for this material is the TNM Classification of Malignant Tumours 7th Edition *(2009) published by John Wiley & Sons Ltd, www.wiley.com.*

CHAPTER 4 | 7th Edition of TNM for Lung and Pleural Tumours

Introductory Notes: The classifications apply to carcinomas of the lung including non-small cell and small-cell carcinoma, broncho-pulmonary carcinoid tumours and malignant mesothelioma of the pleura. Sarcomas and other rare tumours are not included.

Each site is described under the following headings:

- Rules for classification with the procedures for assessing T, N, and M categories; additional methods may be used when they enhance the accuracy of appraisal before treatment
- Anatomical subsites where appropriate
- Definition of the regional lymph nodes
- TNM Clinical classification
- pTNM Pathological classification
- G Histopathological grading where applicable
- Stage grouping
- Summary

Regional Lymph Nodes

The regional lymph nodes extend from the supraclavicular region to the diaphragm. Direct extension of the primary tumour into lymph nodes is classified as lymph node metastasis.

Distant Metastasis

The categories M1 and pM1 may be further specified according to the following notation:

Pulmonary	PUL	Bone marrow	MAR
Osseous	OSS	Pleura	PLE
Hepatic	HEP	Peritoneum	PER
Brain	BRA	Adrenals	ADR
Lymph nodes	LYM	Skin	SKI
Others	OTH		

R Classification

The absence or presence of residual tumour after treatment is described by the symbol R. The definitions of the R classification are:

RX   Presence of residual tumour cannot be assessed

R0   No residual tumour

R1   Microscopic residual tumour

R2   Macroscopic residual tumour

Additional site-specific guidance can be found in Chapters 5 and 6.

LUNG
(ICD-O C34)

Rules for Classification

The changes to the 6th edition are based upon recommendations from the IASLC Lung Cancer Staging Project (1-6).

The classification applies to carcinomas, including non-small cell and small-cell carcinoma (7) and broncho-pulmonary carcinoid tumours (8). There should be histological confirmation of the disease and division of cases by histological type.

Anatomical Subsites

1. Main bronchus (C34.0)
2. Upper lobe (C34.1)
3. Middle lobe (C34.2)
4. Lower lobe (C34.3)

Regional Lymph Nodes

The regional lymph nodes are the intrathoracic nodes (mediastinal, hilar, lobar, interlobar, segmental and sub-segmental), scalene and supraclavicular nodes.

TNM Clinical Classification

T – Primary Tumour

TX   Primary tumour cannot be assessed, or tumour proven by the presence of malignant cells in sputum or bronchial washings but not visualized by imaging or bronchoscopy

T0   No evidence of primary tumour

Tis   Carcinoma in situ

T1   Tumour 3 cm or less in greatest dimension, surrounded by lung or visceral pleura, without bronchoscopic evidence of invasion more proximal than the lobar bronchus (i.e., not in the main bronchus)

     T1a Tumour 2 cm or less in greatest dimension[1]

     T1b Tumour more than 2 cm but not more than 3 cm in greatest dimension

T2   Tumour more than 3 cm but not more than 7 cm; or tumour with any of the following features[2]:

- Involves main bronchus, 2 cm or more distal to the carina
- Invades visceral pleura
- Associated with atelectasis or obstructive pnemonitis that extends to the hilar region but does not involve the entire lung

     T2a Tumour more than 3 cm but not more than 5 cm in greatest dimension

     T2b Tumour more than 5 cm but not more than 7 cm in greatest dimension

T3   Tumour more than 7 cm or one that directly invades any of the following: chest wall (including superior sulcus tumours), diaphragm, phrenic nerve, mediastinal pleura, parietal pericardium; or tumour in the main bronchus less than 2 cm distal to the carina[1] but without involvement of the carina; or associated atelectasis or obstructive pneumonitis of the entire lung or separate tumour nodule(s) in the same lobe as the primary.

T4   Tumour of any size that invades any of the following: mediastinum, heart, great vessels, trachea, recurrent laryngeal nerve, oesophagus, vertebral body, carina; separate tumour nodule(s) in a different ipsilateral lobe to that of the primary.

N – Regional Lymph Nodes

NX   Regional lymph nodes cannot be assessed

N0   No regional lymph node metastasis

N1   Metastasis in ipsilateral peribronchial and/or ipsilateral hilar lymph nodes and intrapulmonary nodes, including involvement by direct extension

N2   Metastasis in ipsilateral mediastinal and/or subcarinal lymph node(s)

N3   Metastasis in contralateral mediastinal, contralateral hilar, ipsilateral or contralateral scalene, or supraclavicular lymph node(s)

M – Distant Metastasis

M0   No distant metastasis

M1   Distant metastasis

      M1a   Separate tumour nodule(s) in a contralateral lobe; tumour with pleural nodules or malignant pleural or pericardial effusion[3]

      M1b   Distant metastasis

Notes: 1. The uncommon superficial spreading tumour of any size with its invasive component limited to the bronchial wall, which may extend proximal to the main bronchus, is also classified as T1a.

2. T2 tumours with these features are classified T2a if 5 cm or less or if size cannot be determined, and T2b if greater than 5 cms but not larger than 7 cms.

3. Most pleural (pericardial) effusions with lung cancer are due to tumour. In a few patients, however, multiple microscopical examinations of pleural (pericardial) fluid are negative for tumour, and the fluid is non-bloody and is not an exudate. Where these elements and clinical judgment dictate that the effusion is not related to the tumour, the effusion should be excluded as a staging element and the patient should be classified as M0.

pTNM Pathological Classification

The pT, pN, and pM categories correspond to the T, N, and M categories.

pN0   Histological examination of hilar and mediastinal lymphadenectomy specimen(s) will ordinarily include 6 or more lymph nodes/stations. Three of these nodes/stations should be mediastinal, including the subcarinal nodes and three from N1 nodes/stations. Labelling according to the IASLC chart and table of definitions given in Chapter 5 is desirable. If all the lymph nodes examined are negative, but the number ordinarily examined is not met, classify as pN0.

G – Histopathological Grading

GX   Grade of differentiation cannot be assessed
G1   Well differentiated
G2   Moderately differentiated
G3   Poorly differentiated
G4   Undifferentiated

Stage grouping

Occult carcinoma	TX	N0	M0
Stage 0	Tis	N0	M0
Stage IA	T1a,b	N0	M0
Stage IB	T2a	N0	M0
Stage IIA	T2b	N0	M0
	T1a,b	N1	M0
	T2a	N1	M0
Stage IIB	T2b	N1	M0
	T3	N0	M0
Stage IIIA	T1a,b, T2a,b	N2	M0
	T3	N1, N2	M0
	T4	N0, N1	M0
Stage IIIB	T4	N2	M0
	Any T	N3	M0
Stage IV	Any T	Any N	M1

TX	Positive cytology only
T1	≤3 cm
T1a	≤2 cm
T1b	>2-3 cm
T2	Main bronchus ≥2 cm from carina, invades visceral pleura, partial atelectasis
T2a	>3-5 cm
T2b	>5 cm-7 cm,
T3	>7 cm; chest wall, diaphragm, pericardium, mediastinal pleura, main bronchus <2 cm from carina, total atelectasis, separate nodule(s) in same lobe
T4	Mediastinum, heart, great vessels, carina, trachea, oesophagus, vertebra; separate tumour nodule(s) in a different ipsilateral lobe
N1	Ipsilateral peribronchial, ipsilateral hilar
N2	Subcarinal, ipsilateral mediastinal
N3	Contralateral mediastinal or hilar, scalene or supraclavicular
M1	Distant metastasis
M1a	Separate tumour nodule(s) in a contra-lateral lobe; pleural nodules or malignant pleural or pericardial effusion
M1b	Distant metastasis

Summary: LUNG

PLEURAL MESOTHELIOMA
(ICD-O C38.4)

Definition of TNM
T - Primary Tumour
T1   T1a   Tumour limited to the ipsilateral parietal pleura with or without mediastinal with or without diaphragmatic pleural involvement

No involvement of the visceral pleura

       T1b   Tumour involving the ipsilateral parietal pleura with or without mediastinal with or without diaphragmatic pleural involvement

Tumour involving the visceral pleura

T2   Tumour involving each of the ipsilateral pleural surfaces (parietal, mediastinal, diaphragmatic, and visceral pleura) with at least one of the following features:

- involvement of diaphragmatic muscle
- extension of tumour from visceral pleura into the underlying pulmonary parenchyma

T3*   Tumour involving all of the ipsilateral pleural surfaces (parietal, mediastinal, diaphragmatic, and visceral pleura) with at least one of the following features:

- involvement of the endothoracic fascia
- extension into the mediastinal fat
- solitary, completely resectable focus of tumour extending into the soft tissues of the chest wall
- non-transmural involvement of the pericardium

T4#   Tumour involving all of the ipsilateral pleural surfaces (parietal, mediastinal, diaphragmatic, and visceral pleura) with at least one of the following features:

- diffuse extension or multifocal masses of tumour in the chest wall, with or without associated rib destruction
- direct transdiaphragmatic extension of tumour to the peritoneum
- direct extension of tumour to the contralateral pleura
- direct extension of tumour to mediastinal organs
- direct extension of tumour into the spine
- tumour extending through to the internal surface of the pericardium with or without a pericardial effusion; or tumour involving the myocardium

N - Regional Lymph Nodes

NX   Regional lymph nodes cannot be assessed

N0   No regional lymph node metastases

N1   Metastases in the ipsilateral bronchopulmonary or hilar lymph nodes

N2   Metastases in the subcarinal or the ipsilateral mediastinal lymph nodes including the ipsilateral internal mammary and peridiaphragmatic nodes

N3   Metastases in the contralateral mediastinal, contralateral internal mammary, ipsilateral or contralateral supraclavicular lymph nodes

M - Distant Metastasis

M0   No distant metastasis

M1   Distant metastasis present

T3 describes locally advanced, but potentially ressectable tumour.
#T4 describes locally advanced, technically unresectable tumour.

Anatomical Stage Groups

Stage I	T1	N0	M0
Stage IA	T1a	N0	M0
Stage IB	T1b	N0	M0
Stage II	T2	N0	M0
Stage III	T1, T2	N1	M0
	T1, T2	N2	M0
	T3	N0, N1, N2	M0
Stage IV	T4	Any N	M0
	Any T	N3	M0
	Any T	Any N	M1

Summary: PLEURAL MESOTHELIOMA

T1	Ipsilateral parietal pleura
T1a	No visceral pleura
T1b	Visceral pleura
T2	Ipsilateral lung or diaphragmatic muscle
T3	Endothoracic fascia, mediastinal fat, focal chest wall or non-transmural pericardium
T4	Contralateral pleura, peritoneum, diffuse or multifocal chest wall, mediastinal organs, myocardium, spine, transmural pericardium or pericardial effusion
N1	Ipsilateral bronchopulmonary or hilar
N2	Subcarinal, ipsilateral mediastinal or internal mammary and peridiaphragmatic
N3	Contralateral mediastinal or internal mammary, ipsilateral or contralateral supraclavicular
M1	Distant metastasis

References:

(1) Goldstraw P, Crowley J, IASLC International Staging Project. The IASLC International Staging Project on Lung Cancer. *J Thorac Oncol 1*, 281-286. 2006.

(2) Rami-Porta R, Ball D, Crowley JJ, Giroux DJ, Jett JR, Travis WD, et al. The IASLC Lung Cancer Staging Project: Proposals for the revision of the T descriptors in the forthcoming (seventh) edition of the TNM classification for lung cancer. *J Thorac Oncol 2*, 593-602. 2007.

(3) Rusch VR, Crowley JJ, Giroux DJ, Goldstraw P, Im J-G, Tsuboi M, et al. The IASLC Lung Cancer Staging Project: Proposals for revision of the N descriptors in the forthcoming (seventh) edition of the TNM classification for lung cancer. *J Thorac Oncol 2*, 603-612. 2007.

(4) Postmus PE, Brambilla E, Chansky K, Crowley J, Goldstraw P, Patz EF, et al. The IASLC Lung Cancer Staging Project: Proposals for revision of the M descriptors in the forthcoming (seventh) edition of the TNM classification for lung cancer. *J Thorac Oncol 2*, 686-693. 2007.

(5) Groome PA, Bolejack V, Crowley JJ, Kennedy C, Krasnik M, Sobin LH, et al. The IASLC Lung Cancer Staging Project: Validation of the proposals for revision of the T, N and M descriptors and consequent stage groupings in the forthcoming (seventh) TNM classification for lung cancer. *J Thorac Oncol 2*, 694-705. 2007.

(6) Goldstraw P, Crowley JJ, Chansky K, Giroux DJ, Groome PA, Rami-Porta R, et al. The IASLC Lung Cancer Staging Project: Proposals for revision of the stage groupings in the forthcoming (seventh) edition of the TNM classification for lung cancer. *J Thorac Oncol 2*, 706-714. 2007.

(7) Shepherd FA, Crowley J, Van Houtte P, Postmus PE, Carney D, Chansky K, et al. The IASLC Lung Cancer Staging Project: Proposals regarding the clinical staging of small-cell lung cancer in the forthcoming (seventh) edition of the TNM classification for lung cancer. *J Thorac Oncol 2*, 1067-1077. 2007.

(8) Travis WD, Giroux DJ, Chansky K, Crowley J, Asamura H, Brambilla E, et al. The IASLC Lung Cancer Staging Project: Proposals for the inclusion of Carcinoid tumours in the forthcoming (seventh) edition of the TNM Classification for Lung Cancer. *J Thorac Oncol 3*, 1213-1223. 2008.

SUPPLEMENTARY INFORMATION AND EXPLANATORY NOTES

Editor's Note: The UICC provides further guidance on the application of the TNM classification in its TNM Supplement: A Commentary on Uniform Use. The sections relating to lung and pleural tumors are reproduced in the next 4 chapters. Chapter 5 provides additional explanatory notes relevant to lung and pleural tumors, Chapter 6 provides specific comments regarding pathological T and N categories, and Chapter 7 contains information on refinements under consideration for future revisions. Their use is recommended to provide the data needed for analysis and validation before possible incorporation in future revisions. Chapter 8 suggests "telescopic ramifications" that could, after data collection, analysis, and validation, amalgamate and simplify classification in future revisions.

Acknowledgment: Used with the permission of the International Union Against Cancer (UICC), Geneva, Switzerland. The original source for this material is the TNM Supplement: A Commentary on Uniform Use, 4th Edition (2009) published by John Wiley & Sons Ltd, www.wiley.com.

CHAPTER 5 | Site-Specific Explanatory Notes for Lung and Pleural Tumours

LUNG

Rules for classification

The classification applies to all types of carcinoma including non-small cell and small cell carcinoma and to broncho-pulmonary carcinoid tumours. It does not apply to sarcomas and other rare tumours.

Changes to the 6th edition are based upon recommendations from the IASLC Lung Cancer Staging Project (1-6).

Clinical classification (Pre-treatment clinical classification), designated TNM (or cTNM), is essential to select and evaluate therapy. This is based on evidence acquired before treatment. Such evidence arises from physical examination, imaging (e.g., computed tomography and positron emission tomography), endoscopy (bronchoscopy or oesophagoscopy, with/without ultrasound directed biopsies [EBUS, EUS]), biopsy (including mediastinoscopy, mediastinotomy, thoracocentesis and video-assisted thoracoscopy), as well as surgical exploration, and other relevant examinations such as pleural/pericardial aspiration for cytology.

Pathological classification (post-surgical histopathological classification), designated pTNM, provides the most precise data to estimate prognosis and calculate end results. This is based on the evidence acquired before treatment, supplemented or modified by the additional evidence acquired from surgery and from pathological examination. The pathological assessment of the primary tumour (pT) entails a resection of the primary tumour, or biopsy adequate to evaluate the highest pT category. Removal of nodes adequate to validate the absence of regional lymph node metastasis is required for pN0. The pathological assessment of distant metastasis (pM) entails microscopic examination.

Pathologic staging depends on the proven anatomic extent of disease, whether or not the primary lesion has been completely removed. If a biopsied primary tumour technically cannot be removed, or when it is unreasonable to remove it, the criteria for pathologic classification and staging are satisfied without total removal of the primary cancer if: a) biopsy has confirmed a pT category and there is microscopical confirmation of nodal disease at any level (pN1-3), b) there is microscopical confirmation of the highest N category (pN3), or c) there is microscopical confirmation of pM1.

General Rule 3 states that clinical and pathological data may be combined when only partial information is available in either the pathological classification or the clinical classification, e.g., the classification of a case designated as cT1 pN2 cM1 or pT2 cN0 cM1 would be considered a clinical classification whilst in a case designated pT2 pN2 cM1, cT2 pN3 cM0 or cT2 cN0 pM1 case it would be appropriate to designate a pathological classification.

Histopathologic Type
(World Health Organization histological classification of tumours of the lung, 2004).

Malignant Epithelial Tumours	ICD#
Squamous cell carcinoma	8070/3
Papillary	8052/3
Clear Cell	8084/3
Small Cell	8073/3
Basaloid	8083/3
Small cell carcinoma	8041/3
Combined small cell carcinoma	8045/3
Adenocarcinoma	8140/3
Adenocarcinoma, mixed subtype	8255/3
Acinar adenocarcinoma	8550/3
Papillary adenocarcinoma	8260/3
Bronchioloalveolar carcinoma	8250/3
Nonmucinous	8252/3
Mucinous	8253/3
Mixed nonmucinous and mucinous or indeterminate	8254/3
Solid adenocarcinoma with mucin production	8230/3

Adenocarcinoma (cont.)	
Fetal adenocarcinoma	8333/3
Mucinous ("colloid") carcinoma	8480/3
Mucinous cystadenocarcinoma	8470/3
Signet ring adenocarcinoma	8490/3
Clear cell adenocarcinoma	8310/3
Large cell carcinoma	8012/3
Large cell neuroendocrine carcinoma	8013/3
Combined large cell neuroendocrine carcinoma	8013/3
Basaloid carcinoma	8123/3
Lymphoepithelioma-like carcinoma	8082/3
Clear cell carcinoma	8310/3
Large cell carcinoma with rhabdoid phenotype	8014/3
Adenosquamous carcinoma	8560/3
Sarcomatoid carcinoma	8033/3
Pleomorphic carcinoma	8022/3
Spindle cell carcinoma	8032/3
Giant cell carcinoma	8031/3
Carcinosarcoma	8980/3
Pulmonary blastoma	8972/3
Carcinoid tumour	8240/3
Typical carcinoid	8240/3
Atypical carcinoid	8249/3
Salivary gland tumours	
Mucoepidermoid carcinoma	8430/3
Adenoid cystic carcinoma	8200/2
Epithelial-myoepithelial carcinoma	8562/3

Morphology code of the International Classification of Diseases for Oncology (ICD-0) and the Systematized Nomenclature of Medicine (www.cap.org). Behavior is coded /0 for benign tumours, /3 for malignant tumours, and /1 for borderline or uncertain behavior. From: Travis WD et al (7). Used with permission.

Summary: LUNG

TX   Primary tumour cannot be assessed, or tumour proven by the presence of malignant cells in sputum or bronchial washings but not visualized by imaging or bronchoscopy

T0   No evidence of primary tumour

Tis   Carcinoma in situ

T1   Tumour 3 cm or less in greatest dimension, surrounded by lung or visceral pleura, without bronchoscopic evidence of invasion more proximal than the lobar bronchus (i.e., not in the main bronchus)

T1a   Tumour 2 cm or less in greatest dimension[1]

T1b   Tumour more than 2 cm but not more than 3 cm in greates dimension

T2   Tumour more than 3 cm but not more than 7 cm; or tumour with any of the following features[2]:

- Involves main bronchus, 2 cm or more distal to the carina
- Invades visceral pleura
- Associated with atelectasis or obstructive pneumonitis that extends to the hilar region but does not involve the entire lung

T2a   Tumour more than 3 cm but not more than 5 cm in greatest dimension

T2b   Tumour more than 5 cm but not more than 7 cm in greatest dimension

T3   Tumour more than 7 cm or one that directly invades any of the following: chest wall (including superior sulcus tumours), diaphragm, phrenic nerve, mediastinal pleura, parietal pericardium; or tumour in the main bronchus less than 2 cm distal to the carina[1] but without involvement of the carina; or associated atelectasis or obstructive pneumonitis of the entire lung or separate tumour nodule(s) in the same lobe as the primary.

T4   Tumour of any size that invades any of the following: mediastinum, heart, great vessels, trachea, recurrent laryngeal nerve, oesophagus, vertebral body, carina; separate tumour nodule(s) in a different ipsilateral lobe to that of the primary.

N – Regional Lymph Nodes

NX   Regional lymph nodes cannot be assessed

N0   No regional lymph node metastasis

N1   Metastasis in ipsilateral peribronchial and/or ipsilateral hilar lymph nodes and intrapulmonary nodes, including involvement by direct extension

N2   Metastasis in ipsilateral mediastinal and/or subcarinal lymph node(s)

N3   Metastasis in contralateral mediastinal, contralateral hilar, ipsilateral or contralateral scalene, or supraclavicular lymph node(s)

M – Distant Metastasis

M0   No distant metastasis

M1   Distant metastasis

M1a   Separate tumour nodule(s) in a contralateral lobe; tumour with pleural nodules or malignant pleural or pericardial effusion[3]

M1b Distant metastasis

Notes: 1. The uncommon superficial spreading tumour of any size with its invasive component limited to the bronchial wall, which may extend proximal to the main bronchus, is also classified as T1a.

2. T2 tumours with these features are classified T2a if 5 cm or less or if size cannot be determined, and T2b if greater than 5 cms but not larger than 7 cms.

3. Most pleural (pericardial) effusions with lung cancer are due to tumour. In a few patients, however, multiple microscopical examinations of pleural (pericardial) fluid are negative for tumour, and the fluid is non-bloody and is not an exudate. Where these elements and clinical judgment dictate that the effusion is not related to the tumour, the effusion should be excluded as a staging element and the patient should be classified as M0.

T Classification

1. Invasion of visceral pleura (T2) is defined as "invasion beyond the elastic layer including invasion to the visceral pleural surface." The use of elastic stains is recommended when this feature is not clear on routine histology (8). See Chapter 7 for additional information.

2. Tumour with direct invasion of an adjacent lobe, across the fissure or by direct extension at a point where the fissure is deficient, should be classified as T2a unless other criteria assign a higher T category.

3. Invasion of phrenic nerve is classified as T3.

4. Vocal cord paralysis (resulting from involvement of the recurrent branch of the vagus nerve), superior vena caval obstruction, or compression of the trachea or esophagus may be related to direct extension of the primary tumour or to lymph node involvement. If associated with direct extension of the primary tumour a classification of T4 is recommended. If the primary tumour is peripheral, vocal cord paralysis is usually related to the presence of N2 disease and should be classified as such.

5. T4: the "great vessels" are
   - Aorta
   - Superior vena cava
   - Inferior vena cava
   - Main pulmonary artery (pulmonary trunk)
   - Intrapericardial portions of the right and left pulmonary artery
   - Intrapericardial portions of the superior and inferior right and left

pulmonary veins

Invasion of more distal branches does not qualify for classification as T4.

6. The designation of "Pancoast" tumour relates to the symptom complex or syndrome caused by a tumour arising in the superior sulcus of the lung that involves the inferior branches of the brachial plexus (C8 and/or T1) and, in some cases, the stellate ganglion. Some superior sulcus tumours are more anteriorly located, and cause fewer neurological symptoms but encase the subclavian vessels. The extent of disease varies in these tumours, and they should be classified according to the established rules. If there is evidence of invasion of the vertebral body or spinal canal, encasement of the subclavian vessels, or unequivocal involvement of the superior branches of the brachial plexus (C8 or above), the tumour is then classified as T4. If no criteria for T4 disease as present, the tumour is classified as T3.

7. Direct extension to parietal pericardium is classified T3 and to visceral pericardium, T4.

8. Tumour extending to rib is classified as T3.

9. The uncommon superficial spreading tumour of any size with its invasive component limited to the bronchial wall, which may extend proximal to the main bronchus, is classified as T1a.

10. The classification of additional tumour nodules in lung cancer depends upon their histological appearances.

    a) In most situations in which additional tumour nodules are found in association with a lung primary these are metastatic nodules, with identical histological appearances to that of the primary tumour. If limited to the lobe of the primary tumour such tumours are classified as T3, when found in other ipsilateral lobes are designated as T4 and if found in the contralateral lung are designated M1a.

    b) Multiple tumours may be considered to be synchronous primaries if they are of different histological cell types. Multiple tumours of similar histological appearance should only be considered to be synchronous primary tumours if in the opinion of the pathologist, based on features such as differences in morphology, immunohistochemistry and/or molecular studies, or, in the case of squamous cancers, are associated with carcinoma in situ, they represent differing sub-types of the same histopathological cell type. Such cases should also have no evidence of mediastinal nodal metastases or of nodal metastases within a common nodal drainage. These circumstances are most commonly encountered when dealing with either bronchioloalveolar carcinomas or adenocarcinomas of mixed subtype with a bronchioloalveolar component. Multiple synchronous primary tumours should be staged separately. The highest T category and stage of disease should be assigned and the multiplicity or the number of tumours should be indicated in parentheses, e.g., T2(m) or T2(5). This distinction may require histopathological confirmation of cell type from more than one tumour nodule, where clinically appropriate.

In the above classification Lung differs from other sites in the application of General Rule 5 as the classification of additional tumour nodules applies not only to grossly recognizable tumours but also those that are microscopic or otherwise only discovered on pathological examination, a not unusual finding in lung cancer.

11. Invasion into mediastinal fat is T4. However, if such invasion is clearly limited to fat within the hilum, classification as T2a or T2b is appropriate, depending upon size, unless other features dictate a higher T category.

N Classification

1. The regional lymph nodes are the intrathoracic, scalene, and supraclavicular nodes.

2. The International Association for the Study of Lung Cancer (IASLC) lymph node definitions are now the recommended means of describing regional lymph node involvement for lung cancers (9) (see Table 5.1). Two versions of the IASLC nodal map have been developed (see Figures 5.1 and 5.2), one pictorial and the other diagrammatic. Both accurately depict the nodal stations defined in the table and show the proposed nodal "zones". Either may be used depending upon preference and the use to which the chart is to be put.

In this nomenclature ipsilateral or contralateral node involvement in #1 would be classified as N3. Involvement of mediastinal nodes, if limited to the midline stations or ipsilateral stations (#2-9), would be classified as N2. Involvement of #10-14 if ipsilateral would be classified as N1. Contralateral involvement of # 2, 4, 5, 6, 8, 9, 10-14 would be classified as N3.

3. Direct extension of the primary tumour into lymph nodes is classified as lymph node metastasis.

Table 5.1. IASLC Nodal Definitions

Nodal station	Description	Definition
#1 (Left/Right)	Low cervical, supraclavicular and sternal notch nodes	Upper border: lower margin of cricoid cartilage Lower border: clavicles bilaterally and, in the midline, the upper border of the manubrium **#L1 and #R1 limited by the midline of the trachea.**
#2 (Left/Right)	Upper paratracheal nodes	2R: Upper border: apex of lung and pleural space and, in the midline, the upper border of the manubrium Lower border: intersection of caudal margin of innominate vein with the trachea 2L: Upper border: apex of the lung and pleural space and, in the midline, the upper border of the manubrium Lower border: superior border of the aortic arch **As for #4, in #2 the oncologic midline is along the left lateral border of the trachea.**
#3	Pre-vascular and retrotracheal nodes	3a: Prevascular **On the right** upper border: apex of chest lower border: level of carina anterior border: posterior aspect of sternum posterior border: anterior border of superior vena cava **On the left** upper border: apex of chest lower border: level of carina anterior border: posterior aspect of sternum posterior border: left carotid artery 3p: Retrotracheal upper border: apex of chest lower border: carina
#4 (Left/Right)	Lower paratracheal nodes	4R: includes right paratracheal nodes, and pretracheal nodes extending to the left lateral border of trachea upper border: intersection of caudal margin of innominate vein with the trachea lower border: lower border of azygos vein 4L: includes nodes to the left of the left lateral border of the trachea, medial to the ligamentum arteriosum upper border: upper margin of the aortic arch lower border: upper rim of the left main pulmonary artery

#5	Subaortic (aorto-pulmonary window)	Subaortic lymph nodes lateral to the ligamentum arteriosum upper border: the lower border of the aortic arch lower border: upper rim of the left main pulmonary artery
#6	Para-aortic nodes (ascending aorta or phrenic)	Lymph nodes anterior and lateral to the ascending aorta and aortic arch upper border: a line tangential to the upper border of the aortic arch lower border: the lower border of the aortic arch
#7	Subcarinal nodes	upper border: the carina of the trachea lower border: the upper border of the lower lobe bronchus on the left; the lower border of the bronchus intermedius on the right
#8 (Left/Right)	Para-esophageal nodes (below carina)	Nodes lying adjacent to the wall of the esophagus and to the right or left of the midline, excluding subcarinal nodes upper border: the upper border of the lower lobe bronchus on the left; the lower border of the bronchus intermedius on the right lower border: the diaphragm
#9 (Left/Right)	Pulmonary ligament nodes	Nodes lying within the pulmonary ligament upper border: the inferior pulmonary vein lower border: the diaphragm
#10 (Left/Right)	Hilar nodes	Includes nodes immediately adjacent to the mainstem bronchus and hilar vessels including the proximal portions of the pulmonary veins and main pulmonary artery upper border: the lower rim of the azygos vein on the right; upper rim of the pulmonary artery on the left lower border: interlobar region bilaterally
#11	Interlobar nodes	Between the origin of the lobar bronchi *#11s: between the upper lobe bronchus and bronchus intermedius on the right *#11i: between the middle and lower lobe bronchi on the right *optional sub-categories
#12	Lobar nodes	Adjacent to the lobar bronchi
#13	Segmental nodes	Adjacent to the segmental bronchi
#14	Sub-segmental nodes	Adjacent to the subsegmental bronchi

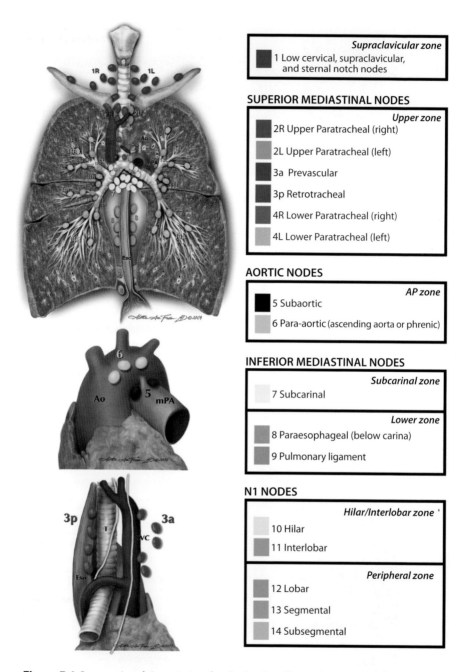

Figure 5.1 International Association for the Study of Lung Cancer Nodal Chart with Stations and Zones. Copyright ©2008 Aletta Ann Frazier, MD.

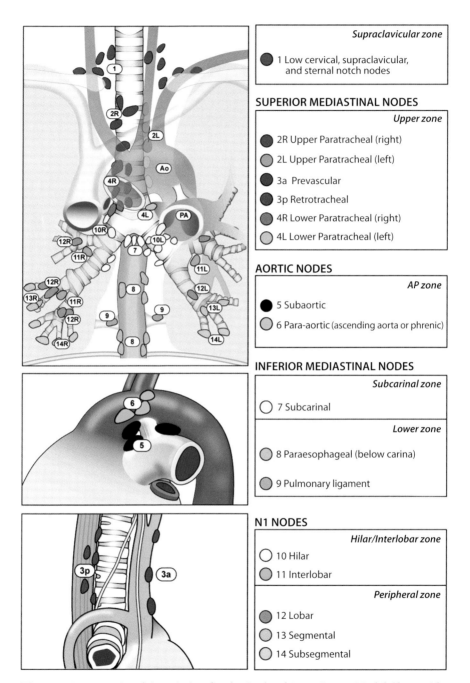

Supraclavicular zone

● 1 Low cervical, supraclavicular, and sternal notch nodes

SUPERIOR MEDIASTINAL NODES

Upper zone

● 2R Upper Paratracheal (right)
● 2L Upper Paratracheal (left)
● 3a Prevascular
● 3p Retrotracheal
● 4R Lower Paratracheal (right)
● 4L Lower Paratracheal (left)

AORTIC NODES

AP zone

● 5 Subaortic
● 6 Para-aortic (ascending aorta or phrenic)

INFERIOR MEDIASTINAL NODES

Subcarinal zone

○ 7 Subcarinal

Lower zone

● 8 Paraesophageal (below carina)
● 9 Pulmonary ligament

N1 NODES

Hilar/Interlobar zone

○ 10 Hilar
● 11 Interlobar

Peripheral zone

● 12 Lobar
○ 13 Segmental
○ 14 Subsegmental

Figure 5.2 International Association for the Study of Lung Cancer Nodal Chart with Stations and Zones. Copyright ©2009 Memorial Sloan-Kettering Cancer Center.

M Classification

1. Pleural/pericardial effusions are classified as M1a.Most pleural (pericardial) effusions with lung cancer are due to tumour. In a few patients, however, multiple microscopical examinations of pleural (pericardial) fluid are negative for tumour, and the fluid is non-bloody and is not an exudate. Where these elements and clinical judgment dictate that the effusion is not related to the tumour, the effusion should be excluded as a staging element and the patient should be classified as M0.
2. Tumour foci in the ipsilateral parietal and visceral pleura that are discontinuous from direct pleural invasion by the primary tumour are classified M1a.
3. Pericardial effusion/pericardial nodules are classified as M1a, the same as pleural effusion/nodules.
4. Separate tumour nodules of similar histological appearance are classed as M1a if in the contralateral lung (vide supra regarding synchronous primaries).
5. Distant metastases are classified as M1b.
6. Discontinuous tumours outside the parietal pleura in the chest wall or in the diaphragm are classified M1b.
7. In cases classified as M1b due to distant metastases it is important to document all of the sites of metastatic disease, whether the sites are solitary or multiple and in addition if the metastases at each site are solitary or multiple.

V Classification

In the lung, arterioles are frequently invaded by cancers. For this reason the V classification is applicable to indicate vascular invasion, whether venous or arteriolar.

Small Cell Carcinoma

The TNM classification and stage grouping should be applied to small cell lung cancer (SCLC). TNM is of significance for prognosis of small cell carcinoma (10), and has the advantage of providing a uniform detailed classification of tumour spread. TNM should be used when undertaking trials in SCLC. The former categories "limited" and "extensive" for small cell carcinoma have been inconsistently defined and used.

Broncho-Pulmonary Carcinoid Tumours

The TNM classification and stage groupings should be applied to carcinoid tumours, typical and atypical variants (11).

Isolated Tumour Cells (ITC)

Isolated tumour cells (ITC) are single tumour cells or small clusters of cells not more than 0.2 mm in greatest dimension that are detected by routine histological stains, immunohistochemistry or molecular methods. Cases with ITC in lymph nodes or at distant sites should be classified as N0 or M0, respectively. The same applies to cases with findings suggestive of tumour cells or their components by nonmorphologic techniques such as flow cytometry or DNA analysis.

The following classification of ITC may be used:

N0   No regional lymph node metastasis histologically, no special examination for ITC

N0(i-)   No regional lymph node metastasis histologically, negative morphological findings for ITC

N0(i+)   No regional lymph node metastasis histologically, positive morphological findings for ITC

N0(mol-) No regional lymph node metastasis histologically, negative nonmorphological findings for ITC

N0(mol+) No regional lymph node metastasis histologically, positive nonmorphological findings for ITC

PLEURAL MESOTHELIOMA

There has been no change in the classification of malignant pleural mesotheliomas from the 6th TNM edition.

1. The staging system applies only to malignant pleural mesothelioma.
2. Regional nodes include: internal mammary, intrathoracic, scalene, and, supraclavicular.

Summary: PLEURAL MESOTHELIOMA

T1   Ipsilateral parietal pleura
    T1a   No involvement of visceral pleura
    T1b   With focal involvement of visceral pleura

T2   Ipsilateral lung, diaphragm, confluent involvement of visceral pleura

T3   Endothoracic fascia, mediastinal fat, focal chest wall, nontransmural pericardium

T4   Contralateral pleura, peritoneum, extensive chest wall or mediastinal invasion, myocardium, brachial plexus, spine, transmural pericardium, malignant pericardial effusion

N1   Ipsilateral bronchopulmonary, hilar

N2   Subcarinal, ipsilateral mediastinal, internal mammary

N3   Contralateral mediastinal, internal mammary, hilar; ipsilateral/
      contralateral supraclavicular, scalene

References:

(1) Goldstraw P, Crowley J, et al. The IASLC International Staging Project on Lung Cancer. *J Thorac Oncol 1*, 281-286. 2006.

(2) Rami-Porta R, Ball D, Crowley JJ, Giroux DJ, Jett JR, Travis WD, et al. The IASLC Lung Cancer Staging Project: Proposals for the revision of the T descriptors in the forthcoming (seventh) edition of the TNM classification for lung cancer. *J Thorac Oncol 2*, 593-602. 2007.

(3) Rusch VR, Crowley JJ, Giroux DJ, Goldstraw P, Im J-G, Tsuboi M, et al. The IASLC Lung Cancer Staging Project: Proposals for revision of the N descriptors in the forthcoming (seventh) edition of the TNM classification for lung cancer. *J Thorac Oncol 2*, 603-612. 2007.

(4) Postmus PE, Brambilla E, Chansky K, Crowley J, Goldstraw P, Patz EF, et al. The IASLC Lung Cancer Staging Project: Proposals for revision of the M descriptors in the forthcoming (seventh) edition of the TNM classification for lung cancer. *J Thorac Oncol 2*, 686-693. 2007.

(5) Groome PA, Bolejack V, Crowley JJ, Kennedy C, Krasnik M, Sobin LH, et al. The IASLC Lung Cancer Staging Project: Validation of the proposals for revision of the T, N and M descriptors and consequent stage groupings in the forthcoming (seventh) TNM classification for lung cancer. *J Thorac Oncol 2*, 694-705. 2007.

(6) Goldstraw P, Crowley JJ, Chansky K, Giroux DJ, Groome PA, Rami-Porta R, et al. The IASLC Lung Cancer Staging Project: Proposals for revision of the stage groupings in the forthcoming (seventh) edition of the TNM classification for lung cancer. *J Thorac Oncol 2*, 706-714. 2007.

(7) Travis WD, Brambilla E, Muller-Hermelink HK, Harris CC. World Health Organisation Classification of Tumours: Pathology and Genetics of Tumors of the Lung, Pleura, Thymus and Heart. Lyon: IARC Press; 2004.

(8) Travis WD, Brambilla E, Rami-Porta R, Vallieres E, Tsuboi M, Rusch V, et al. Visceral pleural invasion: Pathologic criteria and use of elastic stains: Proposals for the 7th edition of the TNM Classification for Lung Cancer. *J Thorac Oncol 3*,1384-1390. 2008.

(9) Rusch V, Asamura H, Watanabe H, Giroux DJ, Rami-Porta R, Goldstraw P, et al. The IASLC Lung Cancer Staging Project: A proposal for a New International Lymph Node Map in the forthcoming (seventh) edition of the TNM Classification for Lung Cancer. *J Thorac Oncol 4*, 568-577. 2009.

(10) Shepherd FA, Crowley J, Van Houtte P, Postmus PE, Carney D, Chansky K, et al. The IASLC Lung Cancer Staging Project: Proposals regarding the clinical staging of small-cell lung cancer in the forthcoming (seventh) edition of the TNM classification for lung cancer. *J Thorac Oncol 2*, 1067-1077. 2007.

(11) Travis WD, Giroux DJ, Chansky K, Crowley J, Asamura H, Jett JR, et al. The IASLC Lung Cancer Staging Project: Proposals for the inclusion of Bronchopulmonary Carcinoid tumours in the forthcoming (seventh) edition of the TNM Classification for Lung Cancer. *J Thorac Oncol 3*,1213-1223. 2008.

CHAPTER 6 | Site-Specific Recommendations for pT and pN Categories

LUNG AND PLEURAL TUMOURS

pT-Primary Tumour

Site	Recommendations
Lung Tumours	The pathologic assessment of the primary tumour (pT) entails resection of the primary tumour sufficient to evaluate the highest pT category (see Chapter 2, General Rule 2b). **pT3 or less** Pathological examination of the primary carcinoma shows no gross tumour at the margins of resection (with or without microscopic involvement). May include additional tumour nodule(s) of similar histological appearance in the lobe of the primary tumour. **pT4** Microscopic confirmation of invasion of any of the following: mediastinum, heart, great vessels, trachea, oesophagus, vertebral body, carina or microscopic confirmation of separate tumour nodule(s) of similar histological appearance in another ipsilateral lobe (not the lobe of the primary tumour).

Site	Recommendations
Pleural Mesothelioma	**pT3 or less** Pathological examination of the mesothelioma with no gross tumour at the margins of resection (with or without microscopic involvement) **pT4** Microscopic confirmation of involvement of the ipsilateral pleural surfaces, with at least one of the following: • Diffuse or multifocal invasion of soft tissues of chest wall • Any involvement of rib • Invasion through diaphragm to peritoneum • Invasion of any mediastinal organ(s) • Direct extension to contralateral pleura • Invasion into the spine • Extension to internal surface of pericardium • Pericardial effusion with positive cytology • Invasion of myocardium • Invasion of brachial plexus

pN - Regional Lymph Nodes

There are no evidence-based guidelines regarding the number of lymph nodes to be removed at surgery for adequate staging. However, adequate N staging is generally considered to include sampling or dissection of lymph nodes from stations 2R, 4R, 7, 10R and 11R for right-sided tumors, and stations 5, 6, 7, 10L and 11L for left-sided tumors. Station 9 lymph nodes should also be evaluated for lower lobe tumors. The more peripheral lymph nodes at stations 12-14 are usually evaluated by the pathologist in lobectomy or pneumonectomy specimens but may be separately removed when sublobar resections (e.g., segmentectomy) are performed. These should be labeled in accordance with the IASLC table of definitions (1) (Table 5.1) and the maps (Figures 5.1 and 5.2) illustrated in Chapter 5.

The UICC recommends that at least 6 lymph nodes/stations be removed/sampled and confirmed on histology to be free of disease to confer pN0 status. Three of these nodes/stations should be mediastinal, including the subcarinal nodes (#7) and three from N1 nodes/stations.

If all resected/sampled lymph nodes are negative, but the number recommended is not met, classify as pN0. If resection has been performed, and otherwise fulfills the requirements for Complete Resection, it should be classified as R0.

Site	Recommendations
Lung Tumours	**pN1** Microscopic confirmation of metastasis in ipsilateral intrapulmonary lymph nodes or ipsilateral peribronchial lymph node(s) or ipsilateral hilar lymph node(s) **pN2** Microscopic confirmation of metastasis in ipsilateral mediastinal lymph node(s) or subcarinal lymph node(s) **pN3** Microscopic confirmation of metastasis in contralateral mediastinal lymph node(s) or contralateral hilar lymph node(s) or scalene or supraclavicular lymph node(s) (ipsilateral or contralateral)
Pleural Mesothelioma	**pN1** Microscopic confirmation of metastasis in ipsilateral bronchopulmonary and/or hilar lymph node(s) **pN2** Microscopic confirmation of metastasis in subcarinal lymph node(s) and/or ipsilateral internal mammary or mediastinal lymph node(s) **pN3** Microscopic confirmation of metastasis in contralateral mediastinal, internal mammary, or hilar lymph node(s and/or ipsilateral or contralateral supraclavicular or scalene lymph node(s)

Site	Recommendations
Lung Tumours	**R1 Microscopic Incomplete Resection** Microscopic evidence of residual disease at any of the following sites: a) Resection margins. b) Extracapsular extension at margins of resecte nodes. c) Positive cytology of pleural/pericardial effusions. **R2 Macroscopic Incomplete Resection** Macroscopic evidence of residual disease at any of the following sites: a) Resection margins. b) Extracapsular extension at margins of resecte nodes. c) Positive nodes not resected at surgery. d) Pleural/pericardial nodules.

If all resected/sampled lymph nodes are negative, but the number recommended is not met, classify as pN0. If resection has been performed, and otherwise fulfills the requirements for complete resection, it should be classified as R0.

Reference:
(1) Rusch V, Asamura H, Watanabe H, Giroux DJ, Rami-Porta R, Goldstraw P, et al. The IASLC Lung Cancer Staging Project: A proposal for a New International Lymph Node Map in the forthcoming (seventh) edition of the TNM Classification for Lung Cancer. *J Thorac Oncol. 4*, 568-577. 2009.

CHAPTER 7 | New TNM Classifications for Testing

a) Concerns have been expressed that the definition of complete resection conferring R0 status is too imprecise and that the application of General Rule 4 does not allow one to assess several features which may represent minimal residual disease and have an adverse prognostic influence. The category "**Uncertain Resection**" has been proposed (1) for testing. There is extant a category "**R1(is)**" which is applicable when the requirements for R0 have been met, but in situ carcinoma is found at the bronchial resection margin. Similarly category "**R1(cy+)**" is appropriate when the requirements for R0 have been met, but Pleural Lavage Cytology (PLC) is positive for malignant cells (v.i.). The wider use of these descriptors is encouraged to facilitate data collection and to assess the prognostic impact of these features following resection. A new category, "**R0(un)**", is proposed to document those other features that fall within the proposed category of "**Uncertain Resection**", i.e., No macroscopic or microscopic evidence of residual disease but any of the following reservations applies:

   i) Nodal assessment has been based on less than the number of nodes/stations recommended for complete resection.
   ii) The highest mediastinal node removed/sampled is positive.

b) A recent meta-analysis (2) has confirmed that pleural lavage cytology (PLC), undertaken immediately on thoracotomy and shown to be positive for cancer cells, has an adverse and independent prognostic impact following complete resection. Such patients may be candidates for adjuvant chemotherapy. Surgeons and pathologists are encouraged to undertake this simple addition to intra-operative staging and collect data on PLC+ve and PLC-ve cases. Where the resection fulfills all of the requirements for classification as a Complete Resection, R0 but PLC has been performed and is positive the resection should be classified as R1(cy+).

c) A standardized definition of visceral pleural invasion (VPI) has been incorporated into the 7th edition of TNM and recommendations included on the use of elastic stains in the determination of VPI (3). It is important that data be collected using this definition so that the utility of this pT2 descriptor can be assessed more accurately in future revisions. A subclassification has been proposed (3) based upon a system published by the Japan Lung Cancer Society (4) and by Hammar (5) (see Figure 7.1). It is proposed that the PL category be used to describe the pathological extent of pleural invasion:

PL0 tumour within the subpleural lung parenchyma or invades superficially into the pleural connective tissue beneath the elastic layer*
PL1 tumour invades beyond the elastic layer
PL2 tumour invades to the pleural surface
PL3 tumour invades into any component of the parietal pleura

*Note: In the TNM 7th edition PL0 is not regarded as a T descriptor and the T category should be assigned on other features. PL1 or PL2 indicate "visceral pleural invasion" i.e., T2a. PL3 indicates invasion of the parietal pleura, i.e., T3.

It is recommended that pathologists prospectively collect data based upon these sub-categories to facilitate future revisions of TNM.

d) There are suggestions that the depth of chest wall invasion may influence prognosis following resection of lung cancer. A sub-classification has been proposed, based upon the histopathological findings of the resection specimen, dividing such pT3 tumours into pT3a if invasion is limited to the parietal pleura (PL 3), pT3b if invasion involves the endothoracic fascia, and pT3c if invasion involves the rib or soft tissue. Pathologists are encouraged to collect this information prospectively to facilitate analysis and future revisions.

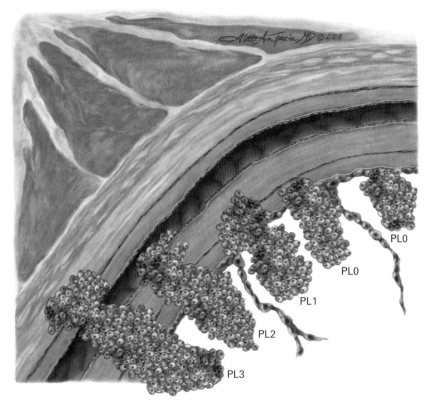

Figure 7.1 Visceral pleural invasion. Copyright ©2008 Aletta Ann Frazier, MD.

e) Imaging evidence of lymphangitis carcinomatosis is usually a contraindication to surgical treatment. The "L" category which is used to assess "lymphatic invasion" is therefore not applicable. The radiological extent of lymphangitis is thought to be of prognostic importance. An exploratory analysis of this feature is proposed using a "cLy" category in which cLy0 indicates that radiological evidence of lymphangitis is absent, cLy1 indicates lymphangitis is present and confined to the area around the primary tumour, cLy2 indicated lymphangitis at a distance from the primary tumour but confined to the lobe of the primary, cLy3 indicates lymphangitis in other ipsilateral lobes and cLy4 indicates lymphangitis affecting the contralateral lung. Radiologists and clinicians are encouraged to collect this information for future analysis.

f) All cases in which there is metastatic spread to distant organs are classified as M1b disease. However, there are clear differences in prognosis based upon tumour burden and the critical nature of some organ sites. Such differences will influence the choice of treatment and the intent of treatment by all modalities of care. Selected patients with isolated metastases to a single organ may benefit from surgical treatment. Clinicians, oncologists and surgeons are encouraged to fully document the extent of disease in M1b cases, collecting data on all of the sites of (suspected) metastatic disease and whether such organs contain single or multiple deposits.

g) The designation of additional tumour nodules of similar histological appearance in the lung(s) has been re-classified in the 7th edition of TNM (6). The UICC cannot determine that this is valid for cases in which multiple deposits are encountered and prospective data collection is necessary to fully validate this re-classification. It is recommended that radiologists, oncologists, surgeons and pathologists document in their clinical and pathological staging the number of nodules in the lobe of the primary, other ipsilateral lobes and the contralateral lung and the diameter of the largest deposit in each location. When found in the lobe of the primary, T3 disease, the size of the closest nodule to the primary tumour and its distance from the primary tumour should also be documented.

h) Carcinoid tumours are included within the 7th edition of TNM. This validates its use by surgeons and pathologists over several decades. However, further details are needed to assess the prognostic impact of certain features in carcinoid tumours (7); Typical versus atypical features, T size cut points, the prognostic impact of multiple deposits and whether these are associated with the syndrome of Diffuse Idiopathic Neuroendocrine Cell Hyperplasia (DIPNECH). In addition, in carcinoid tumours, in which long-term survival can be expected even when associated with multiple tumour nodules or nodal disease, it is important to collect data on disease specific survival. Clinicians, oncologists, surgeons and pathologists are urged to collect such data prospectively.

i) PET scanning using FDG is now widely utilized and has had an impact of the accuracy of clinical staging and referrals for surgical treatment. In addition, a meta-analysis has shown that PET features, such as the maximum value of the Standardized Uptake Value (SUVmax) in the primary tumour prior to treatment is an independent prognostic factor (8). Nuclear medicine specialists, clinicians and oncologists are encouraged to document the use of PET in clinical staging of lung cancer, and to record features such as SUV(max) in the primary and any nodal and/or metastatic sites.

References:

(1) Rami-Porta R, Wittekind C, Goldstraw P. Complete resection in lung cancer surgery:proposed definition. *Lung Cancer* 49, 25-33. 2005.

(2) International Pleural Lavage Cytology Collaborators. Impact of positive pleural lavage cytology on survival in patients undergoing lung resection for non-small cell lung cancer: An international individual patient data meta-analysis. *J Thorac Cardiovasc Surg*. In press, 2009.

(3) Travis WD, Brambilla E, Rami-Porta R, Vallieres E, Tsuboi M, Rusch V, et al. Visceral pleural invasion: Pathologic criteria and use of elastic stains: Proposals for the 7th edition of the TNM Classification for Lung Cancer. *J Thorac Oncol* 3, 1384-1390. 2008.

(4) The Japan Lung Cancer Society. Classification of Lung Cancer: First English Edition. 1 ed. Chiba: Kanehara and Co; 2000.

(5) Hammar SP. Common Tumors. In: Dail DH, Hammar SP, editors. Pulmonary Pathology. 2nd ed. New York: Springer-Verlag; 1994. p. 1138.

(6) Rami-Porta R, Ball D, Crowley JJ, Giroux DJ, Jett JR, Travis WD, et al. The IASLC Lung Cancer Staging Project: Proposals for the revision of the T descriptors in the forthcoming (seventh) edition of the TNM classification for lung cancer. *J Thorac Oncol* 2, 593-602. 2007.

(7) Travis WD, Giroux DJ, Chansky K, Crowley J, Asamura H, Brambilla E, et al. The IASLC Lung Cancer Staging Project: Proposals for the inclusion of Bronchopulmonary Carcinoid tumours in the forthcoming (seventh) edition of the TNM Classification for Lung Cancer. *J Thorac Oncol* 3, 1213-1223. 2008.

(8) Berghmans T, Dusart M, Paesmans M, Hossein-Foucher C, Buvat I, Castaigne C, et al. Primary Tumour Standardized Uptake Value (SUV max) measured on Florodeoxyglucose emission tomography (PDG-PET) is of prognostic value for survival in non-small cell lung cancer (NSCLC): A systematic review and meta-analysis (MA) by the European Lung Cancer Working Party for the IASLC Lung Cancer Staging Project. *J Thorac Oncol* 3, 6-12. 2008.

CHAPTER 8 | Optional Proposals for Testing New Telescopic Ramifications of TNM

The IASLC definitions for individual nodal stations and the resultant nodal charts (see Chapter 5) have been adopted as the new international method for the documentation of nodal stations at clinical or pathological staging where detailed assessment of nodes has been made, usually by invasive techniques or at thoracotomy (1). The concept of nodal zones has been suggested as a simpler, more utilitarian system for clinical staging where surgical exploration of lymph nodes has not been performed (2). An exploratory analysis suggested that nodal extent could be grouped into 3 categories with differing prognoses: i) involvement of a single N1 zone, designated as N1a, ii) involvement of more than one N1 zone, designated as N1b, or a single N2 zone, designated N2a, and iii) involvement of more than one N2 zone, designated as N2b. It is suggested that radiologists, clinicians and oncologists use the classification prospectively, where more detailed data on nodal stations is not available, to assess the utility of such a classification for future revision.

References:
(1) Rusch VR, Crowley JJ, Giroux DJ, Goldstraw P, Im J-G, Tsuboi M, et al. The IASLC Lung Cancer Staging Project: Proposals for revision of the N descriptors in the forthcoming (seventh) edition of the TNM classification for lung cancer. *J Thorac Oncol* 2, 603-612. 2007.
(2) Rusch V, Asamura H, Watanabe H, Giroux DJ, Rami-Porta R, Goldstraw P, et al. The IASLC Lung Cancer Staging Project: A proposal for a New International Lymph Node Map in the forthcoming (seventh) edition of the TNM Classification for Lung Cancer. *J Thorac Oncol* 4, 568-577. 2009.

Editor's Note: The IASLC commissioned Dr. Aletta Frazer to produce a TNM Atlas depicting in pictorial detail each of the T, N and M descriptors. Following a proposal by Drs. Hirokazu Watanabe and Hisao Asamura a CT Atlas was developed depicting the nodal stations on axial, coronal and saggital projections, along the lines of the figures produced by the Japan Lung Cancer Society. The TNM and CT Atlas drawings are depicted here in full color. The colors of the nodal stations in the CT Atlas correspond with those used in the IASLC nodal maps illustrated in Figures 5.1 and 5.2.

CHAPTER 9 | Atlas of Lung Cancer Staging

T1a

T1b

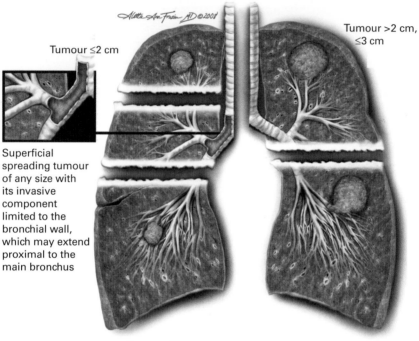

Tumour ≤2 cm

Tumour >2 cm, ≤3 cm

Superficial spreading tumour of any size with its invasive component limited to the bronchial wall, which may extend proximal to the main bronchus

Tumour ≤2 cm; any associated bronchoscopic invasion should not extend proximal to the lobar bronchus

Tumour >2 cm, ≤3 cm; any associated bronchoscopic invasion should not extend proximal to the lobar bronchus

T2a   T2b

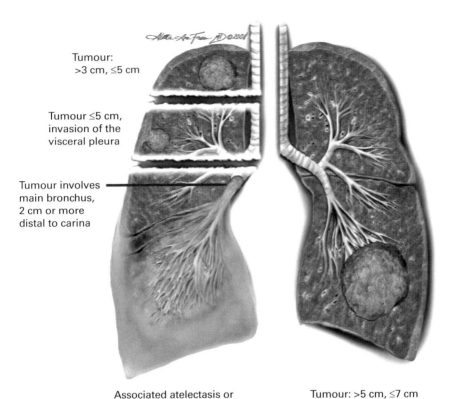

Tumour:
>3 cm, ≤5 cm

Tumour ≤5 cm,
invasion of the
visceral pleura

Tumour involves
main bronchus,
2 cm or more
distal to carina

Associated atelectasis or
obstructive pneumonitis
that extends to the hilar
region but does not involve
the entire lung

Tumour: >5 cm, ≤7 cm
(with or without other
T2 descriptors)

Note: any associated pleural effusion should be shown on multiple
microscopical examinations to be negative for tumour; it should be
non-bloody and not an exudate, and clinical judgement should dictate
that the effusion is not related to the tumour.

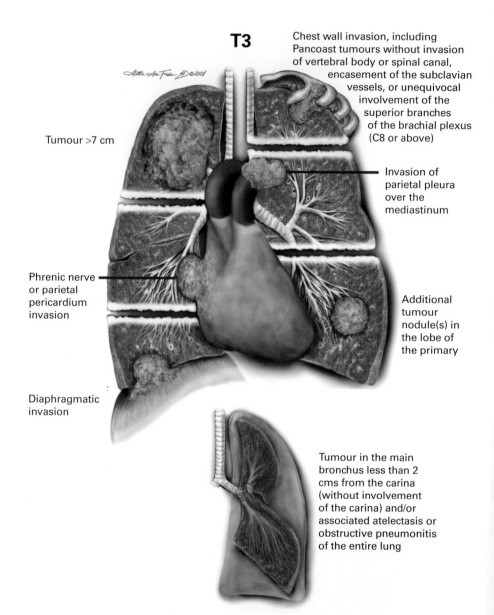

T3

Tumour >7 cm

Chest wall invasion, including Pancoast tumours without invasion of vertebral body or spinal canal, encasement of the subclavian vessels, or unequivocal involvement of the superior branches of the brachial plexus (C8 or above)

Invasion of parietal pleura over the mediastinum

Phrenic nerve or parietal pericardium invasion

Additional tumour nodule(s) in the lobe of the primary

Diaphragmatic invasion

Tumour in the main bronchus less than 2 cms from the carina (without involvement of the carina) and/or associated atelectasis or obstructive pneumonitis of the entire lung

Note: any associated pleural effusion should be shown on multiple microscopical examinations to be negative for tumour; it should be non-bloody and not an exudate, and clinical judgement should dictate that the effusion is not related to the tumour.

T4

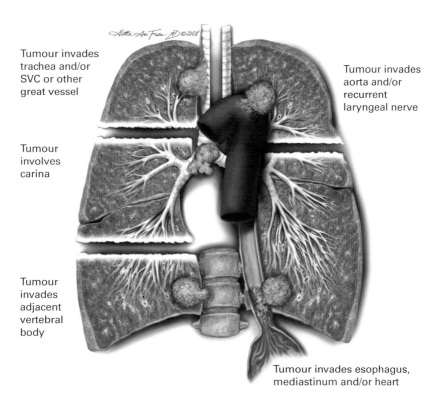

Tumour invades trachea and/or SVC or other great vessel

Tumour invades aorta and/or recurrent laryngeal nerve

Tumour involves carina

Tumour invades adjacent vertebral body

Tumour invades esophagus, mediastinum and/or heart

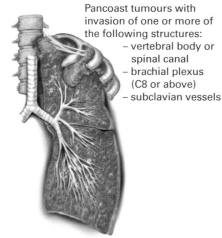

Pancoast tumours with invasion of one or more of the following structures:
– vertebral body or spinal canal
– brachial plexus (C8 or above)
– subclavian vessels

Tumour accompanied by ipsilateral nodules, different lobe

N0   N1

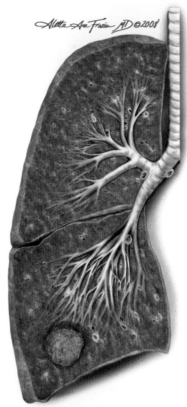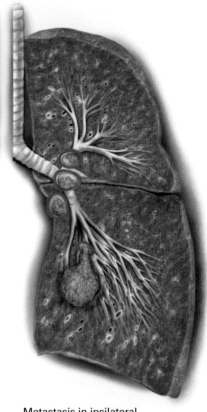

No regional
lymph node
metastases

Metastasis in ipsilateral
intrapulmonary/
peribronchial/hilar lymph
node(s), including nodal
involvement by direct
extension

N2

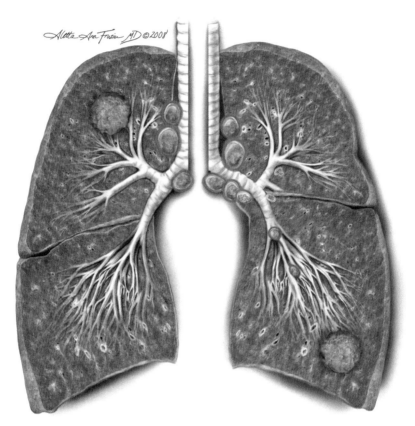

Metastasis in ipsilateral mediastinal and/or subcarinal lymph node(s), including "skip" metastasis without N1 involvement

Metastasis in ipsilateral mediastinal and/or subcarinal lymph node(s) associated with N1 disease

N3

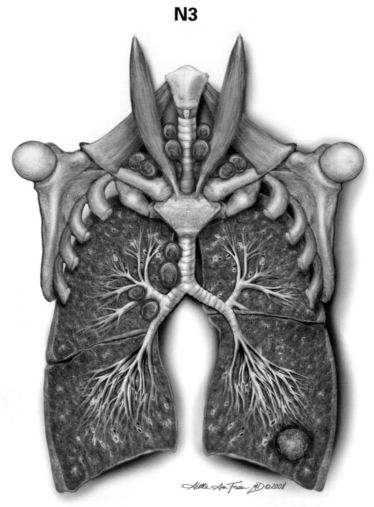

Metastasis in contralateral hilar/mediastinal/scalene/supraclavicular lymph node(s)

Metastasis in ipsilateral scalene/supraclavicular lymph node(s)

M1a

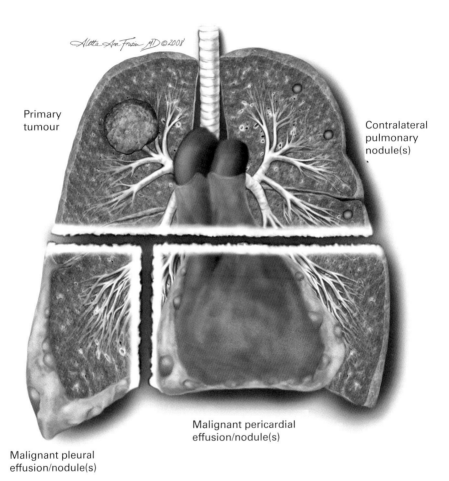

Primary tumour

Contralateral pulmonary nodule(s)

Malignant pericardial effusion/nodule(s)

Malignant pleural effusion/nodule(s)

M1b

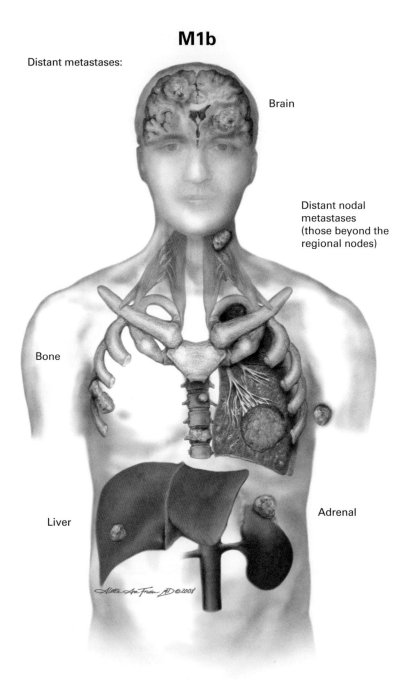

Distant metastases:

Brain

Distant nodal
metastases
(those beyond the
regional nodes)

Bone

Liver

Adrenal

Axial #1

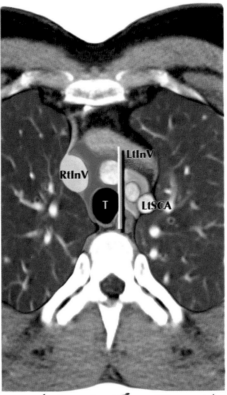

2R 2L

Abbreviations:

Ao – aorta

Az – azygos vein

Eso – oesophagus

InV – innominate vein

LLLB – left lower lobe bronchus

LtInV – left innominate vein

LtMB – left mainstem bronchus

LtPA – left pulmonary artery

LtSCA – left subclavian artery

LtSPV – left superior pulmonary vein

mPA – main pulmonary artery

RtInV – right innominate vein

RtMB – right mainstem bronchus

RtPA – right pulmonary artery

LtPA – left pulmonary artery

SVC – superior vena cava

T – trachea

Axial #2

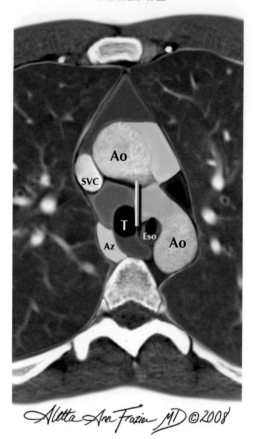

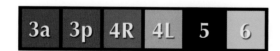

Abbreviations:

Ao – aorta
Az – azygos vein
Eso – oesophagus
InV – innominate vein
LLLB – left lower lobe bronchus
LtInV – left innominate vein
LtMB – left mainstem bronchus
LtPA – left pulmonary artery

LtSCA – left subclavian artery
LtSPV – left superior pulmonary vein
mPA – main pulmonary artery
RtInV – right innominate vein
RtMB – right mainstem bronchus
RtPA – right pulmonary artery
LtPA – left pulmonary artery
SVC – superior vena cava
T – trachea

Axial #3

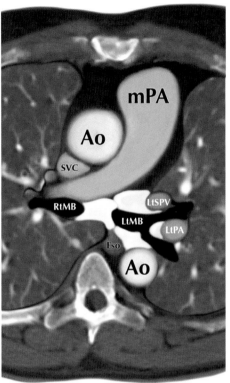

Saggital Left

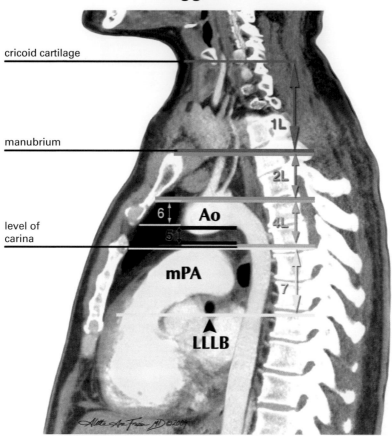

cricoid cartilage

manubrium

level of
carina

1L

2L

6

Ao

4L

5

mPA

7

▲
LLLB

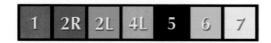

| 1 | 2R | 2L | 4L | 5 | 6 | 7 |

Abbreviations:

Ao – aorta
Az – azygos vein
Eso – oesophagus
InV – innominate vein
LLLB – left lower lobe bronchus
LtInV – left innominate vein
LtMB – left mainstem bronchus
LtPA – left pulmonary artery

LtSCA – left subclavian artery
LtSPV – left superior pulmonary vein
mPA – main pulmonary artery
RtInV – right innominate vein
RtMB – right mainstem bronchus
RtPA – right pulmonary artery
LtPA – left pulmonary artery
SVC – superior vena cava
T – trachea

Copyright ©2008 Aletta Ann Frazier, MD.

Saggital Right

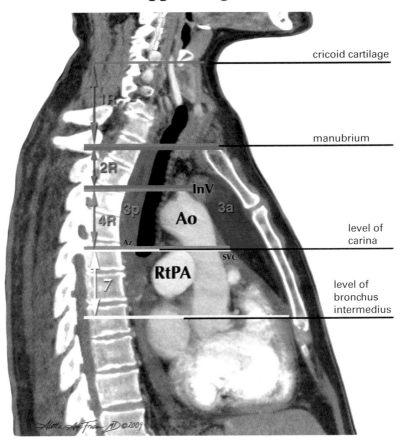

cricoid cartilage

manubrium

level of carina

level of bronchus intermedius

| 1 | 2R | 3a | 3p | 4R | 7 |

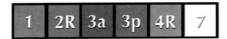
Copyright ©2008 Aletta Ann Frazier, MD.

Coronal

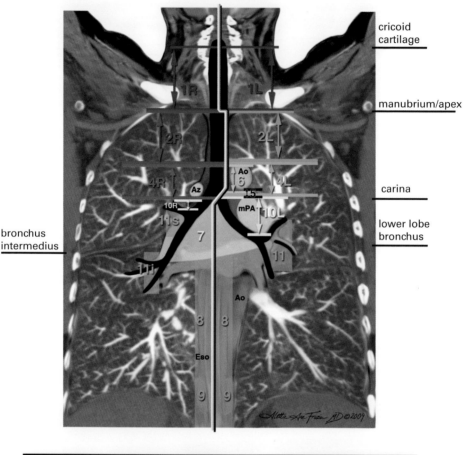

cricoid cartilage

manubrium/apex

carina

lower lobe bronchus

bronchus intermedius

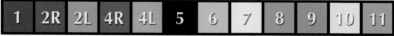

| 1 | 2R | 2L | 4R | 4L | 5 | 6 | 7 | 8 | 9 | 10 | 11 |

Ao – aorta
Az – azygos vein
Eso – oesophagus
InV – innominate vein
LLLB – left lower lobe bronchus
LtInV – left innominate vein
LtMB – left mainstem bronchus
LtPA – left pulmonary artery

LtSPV – left superior pulmonary vein
mPA – main pulmonary artery
RtInV – right innominate vein
RtMB – right mainstem bronchus
RtPA – right pulmonary artery
LtPA – left pulmonary artery
SVC – superior vena cava
T – trachea

Editor's Note: *It was always recognized that the anatomical extent of disease as described by the TNM classification was not the only prognostic factor. Over the years an increasingly large number of rivals have been recognized; tumor-related, patient-related, environmental factors and, recently, molecular markers. Validation for most of these has been incomplete with few population-based studies of sufficient size to allow multifactorial analysis to assess the confounding impact of other factors. This chapter, contributed by the UICC, summarizes the issues raised by these additional prognostic markers and gives guidance as to future research.*

Acknowledgement: *Used with the permission of the International Union Against Cancer (UICC), Geneva, Switzerland. The original source for this material is the Prognostic Factors in Cancer, 3rd Edition (2006) published by John Wiley & Sons Ltd, www.wiley.com.*

CHAPTER 10 | Prognostic Factors: Principles and Applications

Mary K. Gospodarowicz, Brian O'Sullivan, and Eng-Siew Koh

Since the beginning of time, humans have wanted to prognosticate, or "know before". In studies of cancer and other diseases, identification of prognostic factors is the present-day equivalent of predicting the future. Nonetheless, it would be implausible to believe that we can predict precisely for the individual patient. In reality, all we can provide are statements of probability, and even these are more accurate for groups of patients, the study of whom provides us with our knowledge about prognosis. The practical management of cancer patients requires us to make predictions and decisions for individuals, and the challenge of prognostication is to link the individual patient to the collective population of patients with the same disease. The rationale for prognostic factors and classifications of these factors with attention to those used in this book are outlined below. The potential endpoints relevant to oncology, the taxonomy of prognostic factors, and their applications in practice and, most importantly, a concept of a management scenario that forms the basis for defining prognosis at a given point in the course of disease, are presented. The "management scenario" is defined within a specific setting, since prognosis differs for different situations, taking account of the therapeutic milieu, the features of the host and disease, and the particular outcome under study. Prognostic factor research, like clinical trials, must observe essential principles of study assembly and analysis if meaningful conclusions are to be drawn.

RATIONALE FOR PROGNOSTIC FACTORS

The management of patients, or clinical practice, has four main components. Three comprise actions: namely, diagnosis, treatment, and prevention, and one is advisory, that of prognosis. Appraisal of a patient's prognosis is part of everyday practice, and studies of prognostic factors are integral to cancer research. To consider management of an individual cancer case, the fundamental pieces of information required include the site of origin (e.g., lung or breast), and morphologic type or histology (e.g., adenocarcinoma or squamous cell carcinoma).[1-4] In addition, the outcome in a cancer patient depends on a variety of variables referred to as prognostic factors. These factors are defined as variables that can account for some of the heterogeneity associated with the expected course and outcome of a disease. Knowledge of prognostic factors helps us to understand the natural history of cancer. The range of applications for prognostic factors is outlined in Table 10.1.

CLASSIFICATIONS OF PROGNOSTIC FACTORS

There are well-defined and accepted classifications of diseases that include cancer. The best known is ICDO, widely used by cancer registries and administrative bodies. The World Health Organization (WHO) Classification of Tumors forms the basis for the histologic classification in cancer. The TNM classifications published by the International Union

Table 10.1 Application of Prognostic Factors: Learning About the Natural History of Disease

Patient care
• Select appropriate diagnostic tests
• Select an appropriate treatment plan
• Predict the outcome for individual patient
• Establish informed consent
• Assess the outcome of therapeutic intervention
• Select appropriate follow-up monitoring
• Provide patient and caregiver education

Research
• Improve the efficiency of research design and data analysis
• Enhance the confidence of prediction
• Demarcate phenomena for scientific explanation
• Design future studies
• Identify subgroups with poor outcomes for experimental therapy
• Identify groups with excellent outcomes for simplified therapy
• Identify candidates for organ preservation trials

Cancer Control Programs
• Plan resource requirements
• Assess the impact of screening programs
• Introduce and monitor clinical-practice guidelines
• Monitor results
• Provide public education
• Explain variation in the observce outcomes

Against Cancer (UICC) and the American Joint Committee on Cancer (AJCC) are the standard system for recording anatomic disease extent. In contrast to these evidence- and consensus-based agreements, these is no consensus on the optimal classification of prognostic factors. Although no formal system for classifying prognostic factors exists, numerous prognostic indexes and nomograms have been successfully implemented in clinical practice. Previously, we proposed an extremely simple framework for describing prognostic factors in cancer,[2,5] which included the subject-based classification developed to highlight the importance of nontumor related prognostic factors, and clinical relevance classification to highlight the factors indispensable for good clinical practice.

Subject-Based Classification

Most cancer literature equates prognosis with tumor characteristics. Examples include histologic type, grade, depth of invasion, or the presence of lymphnode metastasis. Cancer pathology and anatomic disease extent account for most variations in cancer outcome. However, factors not directly related to the tumor also affect the course of disease and the outcomes of interest. To consider all prognostic factors, we proposed three broad groupings that will be developed further in this edition: those factors that relate to disease or tumor, those that relate to the host or patient, and those that relate to the environment in which we find the patient. In this edition, we focus on prognostic factors that are relevant at the time of diagnosis and initial treatment, although in the management of cancer patients, determination of prognosis is required repeatedly at multiple situations along the course of the disease. These situations often reflect decision-making points, for example, about adjuvant therapy, management of recurrent cancer, and palliative or terminal care

Tumor-Related Prognostic Factors. These include those directly related to the presence of the tumor or its effect on the host, and most commonly comprise those that reflect tumor pathology, anatomic disease extent, or tumor biology (Table 10.2). The fundamental factor to consider is definition of a particular cancer as a distinct disease entity. While histology forms the basis of tumor classification today, the recent revolution in molecular medicine has challenged today's classification and has led to redefinition of many cancers according to molecular and genetic tumor characteristics. These newer criteria have been now accepted in acute leukemia and subtypes of lymphoma. Most new tumor-related molecular factors, such as gene expression patterns, deal with disease characterization.

The second fundamental group of prognostic factors relate to the anatomic extent of disease, so-called "stage," classified according to the UICC TNM classification.[6] In addition to the TNM categories and stage groupings, factors describing disease extent, including tumor bulk, number of involved sites, or involvement of specific organs, and tumor histology, also have an impact on prognosis.[7-10]

Tumor pathology is crucial to the determination of prognosis in cancer. The histologic type has traditionally defined the disease under consideration, but additional factors, such as grade, pattern of growth, immunophenotype, and more recently gene expression patterns, also reflect the fundamental type of disease under consideration. In contrast, multifocality, presence of lymphatic or vascular invasion, infiltration patterns that also affect the outcome may relate both to type of disease and the extent.[11,12] Tumor markers like prostatic-specific antigen (PSA), alpha-feto protein (AFP), and beta human chorionic gonadotropin (HCG) are used in everyday practice and strongly correlate with tumor bulk.[13-15] Hormone receptors, biochemical markers, expression of proliferation-related factors and, increasingly, molecular tumor characteristics that have been shown to affect outcomes for a variety of cancers relate to the type of cancer.[16-18] The presence of symptoms has generally been considered a host factor but it may also be a tumor related factor. A classic example is the presence of B-symptoms (night sweats, fever, and weight loss) in Hodgkin lymphoma.

Table 10.2 Examples of Tumor-Related Prognostic Factors

1. **Pathology**
  Molecular tumor characteristics; gene expression patterns
  Morphologic classification (e.g., adenocarcinoma, squamous)
  Histologic grade
  Growth pattern (e.g., papillary vs. solid, cribriform vs. tubular, vs. solid)
  Pattern of invasion (e.g., perineural, small vessel invasion)

2. **Anatomic tumor extent**
  TNM categories
  Tumor bulk
  Single versus multifocal tumor
  Number of sites of involvement
  Tumor markers (e.g., PSA, AFP, CEA)

3. **Tumor biology**
  Tumor markers (e.g., HER2-neu, CD20)
  Proliferation indices (e.g., S-phase fraction, MiB-1)
  Molecular markers (p53, rb, Bcl2)

4. **Symptoms** (related to the presence of tumor)
  Weight loss
  Pain
  Edema
  Fever

5. Performance status

Host-Related Prognostic Factors. These are factors present in the body of the host (patient) that are not directly related to malignancy, but through interference with the behavior of the tumor or their effect on treatment have the potential to significantly impact the outcome. These factors may generally be divided in demographic patient characteristics, such as age,[19] gender,[20] and racial origin,[21] comorbidity and coexistent illness,[22,23] especially those affecting the immune status,[24] performance status related to comorbid illness, and factors that relate to the host mental state, attitude, and compliance[25,26] with therapy. A history of prior cancer and treatment of that cancer also places survivors at risk for future events (Table 10.3).

Environment-Related Prognostic Factors. The factors that operate external to the patient and could be specific either to an individual patient or, more frequently, to groups of patients residing in the same geographic area. Here, we can consider three categories of environmental factors: first, those that have a physician expertise focus, such as the choice of a specific treatment plan and caregiver skill; second a healthcare system focus including access[27,28] to cancer care, caliber of medical record keeping, internet access,[29] degree of clinical trial participation, and also the presence of ageism, which can all influence treatment selection and outcome. Finally, there are factors related to a society focus, such as a patient's socioeconomic,[30] and nutritional status, and the overall quality of care, including the presence of quality control programs,[31] which may impact the outcome (Table 10.4).

Table 10.3 Examples of Host-Related Prognostic Factors

1. Demographics 　Age 　Race 　Gender 　Level of education 　Socioeconomic status 　Religion
2. Comorbidity 　Constant 　　– Inherited immune deficiency 　　– von Recklinghausen disease, etc. 　Changeable 　　– Coexistent illness (e.g., inflammatory bowel disease, collagen vascular disease) 　– Weight 　– Cardiac status 　– Acquired immune deficiency 　– Infection 　– Mental health
3. Performance status
4. Compliance 　Social reaction to illness 　Influence of habits, drugs, alcohol, smoking, etc. 　Belief in alternative therapies

While a classification within the three subject-based categories may be a useful working model, the distinction between these groupings of prognostic factors is not always clear and many

Table 10.4 Examples of of Environment Related Prognostic Factors

	Related to		
	Treatment	**Education**	**Quality**
Physician	Choice of physician or specialty • Quality of diagnosis • Accuracy of staging Choice of treatment Expertise of physician, "narrow experts" Timeliness of treatment Ageism	Ignorance of medical profession Access to internet Knowledge, education of the patient Participation in clinical trials Participation in continuing education	Quality of treatment Skill of the physician Treatment verification
Health Care System	Access to appropriate diagnostic methods Access to care • Distance • Waiting lists • Monopoly control of access to care Availability of publicly funded screening programs	Continuing medical education Lack of audit of local results Access to internet Development of practice guidelines Dissemination of new knowledge	Quality of equipment Quality management in treatment facility Maintenance of health records Availability of universal health insurance Quality of diagnostic services Implementation of screening programs Promotion of error free environment
Society	Preference for unconventional therapies Socioeconomic status Distance from cancer center Insurance status Access to transportation, car, etc. Ageism	Literacy Access to information	Access to affordable health insurance Nutritional status of the population

prognostic factors overlap these categories. For example, performance status may be related to the tumor, or, when compromised due to coexistent illness, could be a host-related prognostic factor. Similarly, the quality of treatment is a host-related factor if it relates to patient compliance, but is usually an environment-related factor relating to access to optimal medical care. An example of a prognostic factor that fits into all the subject-based categories is anemia[32] and all three could apply to the same patient. Anemia may be a direct result of the presence of tumor mass, as in superficial bladder cancer or cervix uteri cancer, because of persistent heavy bleeding. It may also be a host factor, as in a patient with thalassemia or anemia of chronic disease from an unrelated condition. However, in some parts of the world, as an environmental prognostic factor, anemia also may be a result of malnutrition.

Several prognostic factors, each individually giving predictions with relatively low accuracy, can be combined to provide a single variable of high accuracy. Such a variable is called a prognostic index. Other examples include the International Lymphoma Prognostic Index (IPI)[33] or the Eastern Cooperative Oncology Group (ECOG) performance status scale.

Clinical-Relevance-Based Classification

To consider the relevance of prognostic factors in clinical practice, prognostic factors in this book are placed in three distinct categories: essential, additional, and new and promising factors. Essential factors are those that are fundamental to decisions about the goals and choice of treatment, and include details regarding the selection of treatment modality and specific interventions. In this edition, we have asked the authors to classify as essential exclusively those factors that are required to meet a published clinical practice guideline. This was not possible in all the cases, and as for the other parameters, some variation in the interpretation of the proposed additional factors allow finer prognostication, but are not an absolute requirement for treatment related decision-making processes. Their role is to communicate prognosis, but they do not in themselves influence treatment choice. Finally, our new and promising factors are those that shed new light about the biology of disease, or the prognosis for patients, but for which currently there is, at best, incomplete evidence of an independent effect on outcome or prognosis.

Essential Prognostic Factors. The fundamental factors required to make treatment decision is the type of cancer defined by histology or molecular tumor characteristics. The second most important group of essential factors reflects the anatomic disease extent. The latter has been recognized for over 75 years, when the first attempts at staging classifications were made. Currently, the UICC TNM6 and the AJCC[34] serve to facilitate worldwide communication about cancer. Many other essential factors have been identified including pathology, tumor biology, tumor-related symptoms, patient age, performance status, newer imaging methods,[35-37] and tumor markers[38] are also integral to the decision-making process in the choice of a treatment modality.

Additional Prognostic Factors. In addition to the essential factors, there are numerous variables that help to define the outcome more precisely, but are not required for general decisions about treatment. These include more detailed histologic features, host-related factors, including comorbid conditions and vital organ function, which influence the suitability for surgery, chemotherapy, or radiotherapy. Environment-related factors, such as the choice of an inferior treatment plan, poor quality diagnostic tests, or treatments themselves have the potential to compromise the outcome. Management in a specialized unit,[39] for example, in breast and colorectal cancer, has resulted in improved survival in population-based studies.

New and Promising Prognostic Factors. The immense and rapid expansion of molecular biology has provided an abundance of opportunities to study new biologic prognostic factors,[40,41] which hold promise for future applications. Molecular factors, such as epidermal growth factor receptor (EGFR) status,[42,43] may be used to predict response to a treatment modality, or may present a target for therapy, such as imatinib in gastrointestinal stromal tumors.[44] Alternatively, they may assist in treatment stratification, such as MGMT status, which predicts for chemotherapy and radiotherapy responsiveness in glioblastoma multiforme.[45] Another category includes factors that predict for the presence of occult distant metastases.

A combination of the subject-based and clinical-relevance-based classifications can be used to summarize in simple terms the prognostic factors for individual cancers for a selected management scenario, as depicted in Table 10.5.

Table 10.5 Examples of Prognostic Factors in Cancer

Prognostic Factors	Tumor Related	Host Related	Environment Related
Essential	Anatomic disease extent Histologic type	Age	Availability of access to a radiotherapy facility
Additional	Tumor bulk Tumor maker level	Race Gender Cardiac function	Expertise of a surgeon
New and promising	EGFR (lung, head and neck) Gene expression patterns	Germline p53 mutation	Access to information

MANAGEMENT SCENARIOS: FREEZING THE PROGNOSIS

Since prognosis is a dynamic process affected not only by time, but also other factors, such as the disease and intervention, it is thus useful to apply the concept of *management scenario*, which freezes the prognostic attributes that exist at a given time point, enabling one to then consider how prognosis is influenced by the choice of the planned intervention and the outcome of interest (Fig. 10.1).

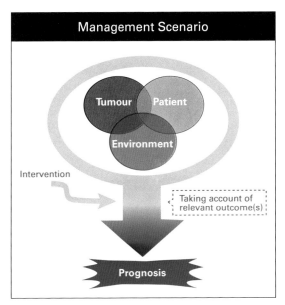

Figure 10.1 Representation of the interaction among the three domains of prognostic factors (tumor, host, and environment). The prognostic factors are express in the context of the proposed therapeutic intervention and for a given endpoint of interest (e.g., survival, response, local tumor control, organ preservation). In addition, the prognosis itself must be interpreted in the context of both the treatment (because it may change the prognosis) and the endpoint (which must be relevant to the prognosis).

For example, in *scenario 1* during a normal physical examination prior to lumpectomy, a patient is found to have a 2-cm breast cancer. Considering the overall survival as the outcome of interest, her prognosis equates to that of reported survival for clinical stage I breast cancer in her peer group (age, race, socioeconomic status) and in geographic region. After the initial treatment is completed, the patient is in *scenario 2*. She has a pT1 pN0 tumor. Her prognosis is better than in scenario 1. She elects to be managed with partial mastectomy alone, her prognosis in scenario 2 is thus less favorable for local control than if she chose to have adjuvant radiation therapy. However, her prognosis for overall survival may not be affected by this decision. After some time, we can construct *scenario 3*. Thus, some years later she develops local recurrence and distant metastasis (scenario 3). Her prognosis for survival is now much worse than in previous scenarios. The progress of time may also affect positively the probability of survival.

Since the prognosis differs with a given scenario, prognostic factors should be considered within a given context or scenario, most commonly before a definitive treatment plan is formulated. Since treatment interventions also have a major impact on the outcome, it is important to discuss prognostic factors in the context of a specific treatment plan or therapeutic intervention.

ENDPOINTS RELEVANT TO CONSIDER IN CANCER PATIENTS

The relevant endpoints to consider in cancer include probability of cure, duration of survival, likelihood of response to treatment, probability of relapse, time to relapse, likelihood of local tumor control, likelihood of organ preservation, and possibility for symptom relief in a palliative context.[46] Therefore, the outcomes may be very heterogeneous. Moreover, some prognostic factors facilitate prediction of more than one outcome, while others predict selected outcomes only.

For example, the presence of bladder muscle wall invasion by a transitional cell carcinoma predicts for distant failure, while its absence virtually eliminates this probability. This knowledge permits clinicians to ignore the possibility of distant failure in patients with superficial bladder cancer both in diagnostic tests and therapeutic interventions. Another example is the number of involved nodal regions in stages I and II Hodgkin's disease that predict for risk of treatment failure, but not for survival. The number of tumors in superficial bladder cancer is predictive for recurrence, but has no impact on the overall survival.

Response to Treatment and Prognosis. Response to treatment is an outcome and as such it always reflects the prognosis. If a response to treatment had no impact on the outcome, such treatment by definition would be ineffective. However, since the knowledge of response is not available until after treatment is initiated, response should not be considered a prognostic factor for the scenario that preceded it.

Tumor response is an early endpoint in the assessment of treatment effectiveness. The four categories of response (complete response, partial response, stable disease, and progressive disease) were originally proposed by the World Health Organization (WHO).[47] Although initially developed to assess the effects of drug therapy, these same criteria may easily be applied to the outcomes of surgical or radiotherapy interventions. For example, complete tumor resection with negative margins could be considered as a complete response to surgical intervention, while positive resection margins could be considered as a partial response to surgical intervention. Thus the extent of response is a surrogate for the anatomic extent of disease after the completion of therapy, and as such is a prognostic factor for further outcome. Since the knowledge of response is not available until after treatment is completed, it should not be considered a prognostic factor for the scenario that preceded it.

TAXONOMY: PROGNOSTIC FACTORS

In the English language, prediction, forecasting, and prognosis all indicate the probability of future events. In medical literature, however, the use of the terms, such as predictive, prognostic, and risk are being freely substituted for each other without much thought about consistent and accurate definitions.

In 1994, Burke[50] proposed that the general heading of predictive factors describe three subtypes: a risk, a diagnostic, and a prognostic factor. In his definition, a risk factor was a factor where the main outcome of interest was incidence and the predictive accuracy was <100%; the diagnostic factor was where the outcome of interest was the incidence and the predictive accuracy was almost 100% of disease. A prognostic factor was where the outcome of interest was death and the predictive accuracy was variable. This classification did not consider the temporal attributes of prediction and is associated with too narrow a view of relevant endpoint for patients with cancer. In epidemiological literature, a risk factor is defined as "a clearly defined occurrence or characteristic that has been associated with the increased rate of a subsequently occurring disease"; thus it is limited to patients who currently do not have a disease. In contrast, a prognostic factor refers to a probability of future event in patients who do currently have a disease.

Henderson and Patek[51] and others defined the term "predictive" as "prognosis for a measurable response" of overt tumor reduction following a treatment intervention and uses the term "predictive factor" as distinct from "prognostic" factor. The authors then consider a prognostic factor in the narrow context of a probability of cure or prolongation of survival. An example of a prognostic factor that is not a predictive factor is the number of involved axillary lymph nodes in breast cancer.[8] A high number of lymph nodes is associated with inferior survival, but the number of involved lymph nodes has no impact on response to treatment. In contrast, a factor that is both predictive and prognostic is the estrogen receptor status in breast cancer that predicts for response to hormonal therapy, but also prognosticates for a better survival. It is debatable whether such a distinction in terminology, which focuses on a single intermediate outcome (a measurable response to cytotoxic treatment) instead of defined endpoint relating to overall prognosis (e.g., local tumor control, survival), should be embraced.

Examples of clinical situations where response is not an indication for the use of treatment include: chemotherapy in an asymptomatic patient with Stage III follicular small-cell lymphoma; androgen deprivation therapy in an asymptomatic patient with Tl prostate cancer; and radiation therapy in stage IV Hodgkin's lymphoma.

Surrogate Diagnostic Factors versus Prognostic Factors. With better understanding of the mechanisms by which prognostic factors predict the future, new endpoints other than long-term survival have emerged. For example, the forecasting of the probability of occult distant metastasis allows for a better understanding of the pattern of failure and targeting of treatment efforts. Where the probability of the presence of occult metastatic disease at the time of diagnosis is concerned, however, these factors predict for the current state and not for a future event. Two examples of such factors are the PSA level[13] and the Gleason score in localized prostate cancer, which are considered as prognostic when survival or treatment failure probabilities are the endpoints of interest, but seen as surrogate diagnostic factors when they help discriminate different states at the present time. The reason is that they may help determine the probability of the presence of subclinical disease (e.g., disease lymph-node involvement) as an endpoint of interest.

Time-Dependent Prognostic Factors. Time-dependent prognostic factors are variables that become available over the time course of the patient's disease. While they may be very predictive of outcome, they are also problematic because they risk disturbing the context of relevant disease outcome evaluation and decision making.[52] This is because it may be impossible to separate real "causality" in the relationship between a time-dependent factor and an outcome of interest from a mere "association" caused by another factor common to them both. Therefore, if not undertaken carefully, the clinical interpretation of time-dependent prognostic factors may be incorrect. In some cases, prognostic factors associated with a subsequent scenario have been considered together with prognostic factors at diagnosis. For example, the postradiotherapy PSA nadir level has been included in Cox models of prognostic factors in localized prostate cancer. In truth, the PSA nadir is a surrogate for response to radiotherapy,[13] and as such belongs to a different management scenario occurring subsequently.

APPLICATION OF PROGNOSTIC FACTORS

Prognostic factors are used in daily clinical practice, in research, and in cancer control. In everyday clinical practice, the influence of prognostic factors dominates all the steps in decision making and the comprehensive management of patients with cancer, including selection of the primary goal of management, the most appropriate treatment modality, and the adjustment of treatment according to disease severity. Knowledge of prognostic factors allows clinicians to select treatment options that allow preservation of organs or function without compromising cure and survival.

The implementation of evidence-based clinical practice guidelines[53] will also serve to improve the quality of decision making and in turn the outcomes in cancer patients. It is thus necessary to know the prognostic factors in a relevant context in order to evaluate compliance with such guidelines to then examine their impact.

Prognostic Factors and Milieu

The prognostic factors that are defined as essential for decision making depend on their relevance to the issues in cancer care in a particular milieu, that is, the practice of cancer care in the first world or conversely in developing countries,[54] where the main issues are related to cancer prevention and early detection. Factors that predict for organ preservation and those that contribute to finesse in defining the prognosis may not be important in places with limited diagnostic equipment, and where funding for evaluation of assessment of response to treatment is not available. The milieu where the patient and healthcare professional are located thus impacts on the interplay of essential, additional, and new and promising factors. Moreover, progress in such situations does not require new discovery, but rather economic development, education, and a continued process to ensure improved access.

FUTURE RESEARCH INTO PROGNOSTIC FACTORS

To be relevant to the clinical practice, prognostic factors must either have a significant impact on cancer outcome, or be used to select treatment methods. It is likely that with progress in treatment, and improved outcomes, prognostic factors will be more relevant for selection of treatment. However, knowledge of prognostic factors is also required to minimize the impact of treatment. Improved staging methods, and especially more accurate characterization of microscopic disease extent will allow a more homogeneous grouping of patients with similar disease characteristics, and the tumor-related prognostic factors for an individual disease may change. Knowledge of genetic factors will further add to the improved prediction of outcome and greater individualization of therapeutic interventions. However, grouping of patients into similar categories will continue to be required to assess the impact of new technology of patient assessment and new therapies on the outcome.

References:

1. Byar D: Identification of prognostic factors, in Buyse ME SM, Sylvester RJ (eds.): Cancer clinical trials. New York: Oxford University Press, 1984, pp. 423-443.

2. Gospodarowicz M, O'Sullivan B: Prognostic Factors: Principles and Application, in Gospodarowicz M, Henson DE, Hutter RVP, et al. (eds.): Prognostic Factors in Cancer. 2nd ed. New York; Wiley-Liss, 2001, pp. 17-36.

3. Stockier M, Tannock I: Guide to studies of diagnostic tests, prognostic factors, and treatments, in Tannock I, Hill, R. (eds.): The basic science of oncology, 3rd ed. Toronto; McGraw-Hill, 1998, pp. 466-492.

4. Riley RD, Abrams KR, Sutton AJ, et al.: Reporting of prognostic markers: current problems and development of guidelines for evidence-based practice in the future. Br J *Cancer* 88:1191-1198,2003.

5. Gospodarowicz M, O'Sullivan, B, Bristow, et al.: Host, and Environment-related Prognostic Factors, in Gospodarowicz M, Henson DE, Hutter RVP et al. (eds.): Prognostic Factors in Cancer, 2nd ed. New York; Wiley-Liss, 2001, pp. 71-94.

6. Sobin LH WC: TNM classification of malignant tumors. 6th ed. New York; Wiley-Liss, 2002.

7. Schmoll HI, Souchon R, Krege S, et al.: European consensus on diagnosis and treatment of germ cell cancer: a report of the European Germ Cell Cancer Consensus Group (EGCCCG), *Ann Oncol* 15:1377-1399, 2004.

8. Truong PT, Berthelet E, Lee I, et al.: The prognostic significance of the percentage of positive/dissected axillary lymph nodes in breast cancer recurrence and survival in patients with one to three positive axillary lymph nodes. *Cancer* 103:2006-2014, 2005.

9. Compton CC: Colorectal carcinoma: diagnostic, prognostic, and molecular features. *Mod Pathol* 16:376-388,2003.

10. Berglund M, Thunberg U, Amini RM, et al.: Evaluation of immunophenotype in diffuse large B-celllymphoma and its impact on prognosis. *Mod Pathol* 18:1113-1120, 2005.

11. Baak IP, van Diest PI, Voorhorst FI, et al.: Prospective multicenter validation of the independent prognostic value of the mitotic activity index in lymph node-negative breast cancer patients younger than 55 years. *I Clin Oncol* 23: 5993-6001, 2005.

12. Truong PT, Yong CM, Abnousi F, et al.: Lymphovascular invasion is associated with reduced locoregional control and survival in women with node-negative breast cancer treated with mastectomy and systemic therapy. *I Am Coll Surg* 200:912-921, 2005.

13. D'Amico AV, Renshaw AA, Sussman B, et al.: Pretreatment PSA velocity and risk of death from prostate cancer following external beam radiation therapy. *IAMA* 294:440-447, 2005.

14. Gorog D, Regoly-Merei I, Paku S, et al.: Alpha-fetoprotein expression is a potential prognostic marker in hepatocellular carcinoma. World I *Gastroenterol* 11:5015-5018, 2005.

15. Paramasivam S, Tripcony L, Crandon A, et al.: Prognostic importance of pre-operative CA-125 in International Federation of Gynecology and Obstetrics stage I epithelial ovarian cancer: an Australian multicenter study. *I Clin Oncol* 23:5938-5942, 2005.

16. DiGiovanna MP, Stem DF, Edgerton SM, et al.: Relationship of epidermal growth factor receptor expression to ErbB-2 signaling activity and prognosis in breast cancer patients. *I Clin Oncol* 23:1152-1160, 2005.

17. Wang Y, Klijn IG, Zhang Y, et al.: Gene-expression profiles to predict distant metastasis of lymph-node-negative primary breast cancer. *Lance*t 365:671-679, 2005.

18. Buscarini M, Quek ML, Gill P, et al.: Molecular prognostic factors in bladder cancer. RIU lnt 95:739-742,2005.

19. HurriaA, Leung D, Trainor K, et al.: Factors influencing treatment patterns of breast cancer patients age 75 and older. *Crit Rev Oncol Hematol* 46:l2l-l26, 2003.

20. Batevik R, Grong K, Segadal L, et al.: The female gender has a positive effect on survival independent of background life expectancy following surgical resection of primary non small cell lung cancer: a study of absolute and rela-tive survival over 15 years. *Lung Cancer* 47:173-181, 2005.

21. Chlebowski RT, Chen Z, Anderson GL, et al.: Ethnicity and breast cancer: factors influencing differences in incidence and outcome. *I Natl Cancer lnst* 97:439-448, 2005.

22. Maas HA, Kruitwagen RF, Lemmens VE, et al.: The influence of age and co-morbidity on treatment and prognosis of ovarian cancer: a population-based study. *Gynecol Oncol* 97:104-109,2005.

23. Ianssen-Heijnen ML, van Spronsen DI, Lemmens VE, et al.: A population-based study of severity of comorbidity among patients with non-Hodgkin's lymphoma: prognostic impact independent ofInternational Prognostic Index. *Rr I Haematol* 129:597-606, 2005.

24. Straus DJ: Prognostic factors in the treatment of human immunodeficiency virus associated non-Hodgkin's lymphoma. Recent Results *Cancer Res* 159: 143-148, 2002.

25. Verkooijen HM, Fioretta GM, Rapiti E, et al.: Patients' refusal of surgery strongly impairs breast cancer survival. *Ann Surg* 242:276-280, 2005.

26. Cathcart CS, DunicanA, Halpern IN: Patterns of delivery of radiation therapy in an innercity population of head and neck cancer patients: an analysis of compliance and end results. *J Med* 28:275-284, 1997.

27. Mackillop WJ, Zhang-Salomons J, Groome PA, et al.: Socioeconomic status and cancer survival in Ontario. *J Clin Oncol* 15:1680-1689, 1997.

28. Jemal A, Ward E, Wu X, et al.: Geographic patterns of prostate cancer mor-tality and variations in access to medical care in the United States. *Cancer Epidemiol Biomarkers Prev* 14:590-595,2005.

29. Till JE, Phillips RA, Jadad AR: Finding Canadian cancer clinical trials on the Internet: an exploratory evaluation of online resources. *CMAJ* 168: 1127-1129, 2003.

30. Freeman HP: Poverty, culture, and social injustice: determinants of cancer disparities. *CA Cancer J Clin* 54:72-77, 2004.

31. Sauven P, Bishop H, Patnick J, et al.: The National Health Service Breast Screening Programme and British Association of Surgical Oncology audit of quality assurance in breast screening 1996-2001. *Br J Surg* 90:82-87, 2003.

32. Munstedt K, Johnson P, Bohlmann MK, et al.: Adjuvant radiotherapy in carcinomas of the uterine cervix: the prognostic value of hemoglobin levels. *Int J Gynecol Cancer* 15:285-291, 2005.

33. Hermans J, Krol AD, van Groningen K, et al.: International Prognostic Index for aggressive non-Hodgkin's lymphoma is valid for all malignancy grades. *Blood* 86:1460-1463,1995.

34. AJCC Cancer Staging Manual. 6th ed.: Springer-Verlag, 2002.

35. Borst GR, Belderbos JS, Boellaard R, et al.: Standardised FDG uptake: a prognostic factor for inoperable non-small cell lung cancer. *Eur J Cancer* 41:1533-1541, 2005.

36. Hutchings M, Mikhaeel NG, Fields PA, et al.: Prognostic value of interim FDG-PET after two or three cycles of chemotherapy in Hodgkin lymphoma. *Ann Oncol* 16: 1160-1168, 2005.

37. Jackson AS, Parker CC, Norman AR, et al.: Tumor staging using magnetic resonance imaging in clinically localised prostate cancer: relationship to biochemical outcome after neo-adjuvant androgen deprivation and radical radiotherapy. *Clin Oncol* (R Coll Radiol)17: 167-171,2005.

38. Lam JS, Shvarts 0, Leppert JT, et al.: Renal cell carcinoma 2005: new frontiers in staging, prognostication and targeted molecular therapy. *J Urol* 173:1853-1862, 2005.

39. Smith ER, Butler WE, Barker FG, 2nd: Craniotomy for resection of pediatric brain tumors in the United States, 1988 to 2000: effects of provider caseloads and progressive centralization and specialization of care. *Neurosurgery* 54:553-563; discussion 56 3-555, 2004.

40. Poon RT, Fan ST, Wong J: Clinical significance of angiogenesis in gastrointestinal cancers: a target for novel prognostic and therapeutic approaches. *Ann Surg* 238:9-28, 2003.

41. Russo A, Bazan V, lacopetta B, et al.: The TP53 Colorectal Cancer International Collaborative Study on the Prognostic and Predictive Significance of p53 Mutation: Influence of Tumor Site, Type of Mutation, and Adjuvant Treatment. *J Clin Oncol* 23:7518-7528, 2005.

42. Shepherd FA, Rodrigues Pereira J, Ciuleanu T, et al.: Erlotinib in previously treated non small-cell lung cancer. *N Engl J Med* 353:123-132, 2005.

43. Bentzen SM, Atasoy BM, Daley FM, et al.: Epidermal growth factor receptor expressionin pretreatment biopsies from head and neck squamous cell carcinoma as a predictive factor for a benefit from accelerated radiation therapy in a randomized controlled trial. *J Clin Oncol* 23:5560-5567, 2005.

44. Van Glabbeke M, Verweij J, Casali PG, et al.: Initial and late resistance to imatinib in advanced gastrointestinal stromal tumors are predicted by

different prognostic factors: a European Organisation for Research and Treatment of Cancer-Italian Sarcoma GroupAustralasian Gastrointestinal Trials Group study. *J Clin Oncol* 23:5795-5804, 2005.

45. Hegi ME, Diserens AC, Gorlia T, et al.: MGMT gene silencing and benefit from temozolomide in glioblastoma. *N Engl J Med* 352:997-1003, 2005.

46. Toscani P, Brunelli C, Miccinesi G, et al.: Predicting survival in terminal cancer patients: clinical observation or quality-of-life evaluation? *Palliat Med* 19:220-227, 2005.

47. WHO handbook for reporting results of cancer treatment, Geneva: World Health Organization Offset Publication, 1979.

48. Zagars GK, Ballo MT, Pisters PW, et al.: Surgical margins and reresection in the managementof patients with soft tissue sarcoma using conservative surgery and radiation therapy. *Cancer* 97:2544-2553, 2003.

49. Smitt MC, Nowels K, Carlson RW, et al.: Predictors of reexcision findings and recurrence after breast conservation.Int J Radiat Oncol BioI Phys 57:979-985, 2003.

50. Burke HB: Increasing the power of surrogate endpoint biomarkers: the aggregation of predictive factors. *J Cell Biochem Suppl* 19:278-282, 1994.

51. Henderson IC, PatekAJ: The relationship between prognostic and predictive factors in the management of breast cancer. *Breast Cancer Res Treat* 52:261-288, 1998.

52. McShane LM, Altman DG, Sauerbrei W, et al.: Reporting recommendations for tumor marker prognostic studies (REMARK). *J Natl Cancer Inst* 97: II 80-II 84, 2005.

53. Woolf SH: Evidence-based medicine and practice guidelines: an overview. *Cancer Control* 7:362-367, 2000.

54. Magrath I, Shanta V, Advani S, et al.: Treatment of acute lymphoblastic leukaemia incountries with limited resources; lessons from use of a single protocol in India over a twenty year period. *Eur J Cancer* 41:1570-1583,2005.

Editor's Note: The scene having been set in the previous chapter the next incorporates site-specific guidance on the present situation regarding additional prognostic factors in several thoracic malignancies; lung cancer, malignant pleural mesothelioma and malignant thymoma. At the end of the lung cancer section we have inserted information on the role of those additional prognostic factors in non-small cell and small cell lung cancer available in the clinically staged, cTNM, and pathologically staged, pTNM, cases within the IASLC International data base. This appendix also contains the summary of a literature review into the present position of biological markers as prognostic indicators.

Acknowledgement: Used with the permission of the International Union Against Cancer (UICC), Geneva, Switzerland. The original source for this material is the Prognostic Factors in Cancer, 3rd Edition (2006) published by John Wiley & Sons Ltd, www.wiley.com.

CHAPTER 11 | Prognostic Factors in Thoracic Malignancies

LUNG CANCER

Michael D. Brundage and William J. Mackillop

Lung cancer is a group of heterogeneous clinical entities with common molecular and cellular origins, but with different accumulated genetic mutations with different clinical behaviors and prognoses. Lung cancers are the most common cause of cancer death in both males and females in North America.[1] A substantive amount of clinical and basic science research has focussed on prognostic factors in patients with lung cancer, and more than 100 prognostic factors pertaining to the tumor, the patient, or the environment having been reported; the reader is referred to more detailed descriptions of the breadth of this literature.[2,3]

The recognized clinical heterogeneity among lung cancer patients has led to the division of prognostic subgroups. The most important distinction is between small cell lung cancer (SCLC) and nonsmall cell lung cancer (NSCLC). The second is disease extent, or anatomical stage. NSCLC, is staged using the TNM classification;[4] SCLC as either limited or extensive disease.[4] Some advocate TNM system for SCLC.[5] A comprehensive review of all prognostic factors is beyond the scope of this chapter, which focuses on those factors that have established clinical relevance to treatment guidelines for these common presentations.[2]

Most studies of NSCLC evaluate patients with resected disease, but few have addressed the prognosis based on preoperative information.[2] In patients with resectable disease, but who are inoperable for medical reasons and treated with radical radiotherapy,[1] T category, symptoms, performance status, and hemoglobin are significant predictors of survival. For patients undergoing resection, with recurrence rates of 20-85%,[4] the determination of prognosis is clinically relevant. Completely resected cases[5] with pT2pNO disease are candidates for chemotherapy, whereas those with pN2 disease or positive resection margins (Rl cases) are candidates for radiotherapy with or without chemotherapy.[1,6] Controversy exists regarding the definition of TNM stage groupings, methods of anatomical staging (including the use of positron emission tomography (PET) scanning),[7-9] and the appropriate extent of mediastinal dissection,[1,3] among others.

The significance of cell type (large-cell undifferentiated, adenocarcinoma, or squamous cell) has been studied extensively. Studies show inconsistent evidence regarding the significance of adenocarcinoma compared to other NSCLC subtypes.[2] Bronchioalveolar cancer and carcinoid tumors constitute notable exceptions.[1] Many other tumor factors have been shown to have independent prognostic significance,[2] but are not utilized routinely for treatment decision making. These factors include histologic features, chemistry, and serum tumor markers, tumor proliferation, and cellular markers. Other molecular markers, include regulators of cellular growth (kRAS, RB, EGFr, erb-b2, MRP-1, HGF), of the metastatic cascade (TPA, Cyclin D-1, cathepsin), and of apoptosis (p53, bcl-2).[1-3,10] Patient-related characteristics predictive after complete surgical resection are less powerful in the setting of resected disease than in the advanced-disease setting. Thus, patient-related factors are generally not considered important for clinical decision making in this scenario, with the exception of comorbidities influencing medical operability and radiotherapy tolerance.[3,4]

The majority of studies consider both locally advanced (typically T4 or N3 or uresectable T3N2 cases) and metastatic NSCLC (M1 cases) under the term of "advanced" disease. The distinction between the two entities, however, is important for the consideration of particular subgroups of patients due to treatment decision-making implications.[1] Factors essential to decision making are stage, weight loss, and performance status, indicators of potential success with combined-modality loco-regional therapy.

Patients without systemic manifestations of illness, those patients with no substantial weight loss, and high performance status, have been shown to have higher survival rates following induction chemotherapy followed by radiotherapy, or concurrent chemo-radiotherapy. They have been shown to have better survival when treated with continuous hyperfractionated and accelerated radiotherapy (CHART) as compared to conventional fractionation, and with higher radiation dose. The role of surgery is currently being investigated, as is the role of combination chemo-radiotherapy in more symptomatic patients.[1] A subgroup of patients is that with cT3NOMO disease, particularly when located in the superior pulmonary sulcus (Pancoast's tumor).[11]

In the setting of advanced (stage IV) disease, markers of functional impact, such as weight loss, performance status, symptom burden, and pretreatment quality of life, have been shown to have independent prognostic significance for median survival duration following systemic therapy. Chemotherapy itself, as an environment-related factor, is known to improve patients' median survival over best-supportive care alone in patients without substantial systemic manifestations of illness. More recent clinical trials research has been directed at finding chemotherapy regimens with higher response rates and/or lower toxicity.[1] Additional factors include markers relating to the extent of clinically detectable disease, hematological or biochemical markers associated with disease extent. In a large study of 2531 patients enrolled on a variety of clinical trials, Albain and colleagues[4] identified good performance status, female gender, and age >70 years as the most important factors for survival overall. Patient self-reported indices, such as quality of life scores and/or anxiety and depression measures, are new emerging prognostic factors.[2]

In the setting of small cell lung cancer (SCLC), stage is considered an essential factor since patients with limited disease generally receive loco-regional radiotherapy and prophylactic cranial radiotherapy in addition to chemotherapy,[1] and are considered potentially curable. The use of prophylactic cranial radiotherapy predicts for fewer central nervous system (CNS) recurrences compared to untreated patients, but has not been consistently shown to increase patients' median survival. The use of loco-regional radiotherapy, in contrast, has been clearly demonstrated to improve survival of limited stage patients. In addition, the timing of thoracic radiotherapy (early vs. late in relation to chemotherapy treatment[12]), and the use of altered fractionation strategies and/or higher doses of radiotherapy have been shown in some studies to increase patient survival. These issues, in addition to novel systemic therapeutic strategies, continue to be investigated in clinical trials.[1] Large studies of treated patient cohorts, have shown outcome in limited disease to be best predicted by good performance status, female sex, age <70 years, white race, normal serum lactate dehydrogenase (LDH), and concurrent chemo-radiotherapy. A normal serum LDH, multidrug chemotherapy, and a single metastatic lesion best predicted survival outcomes for patients with extensive disease.

Table 11.1 Prognostic Factors in Surgically Resected NSCLC

Prognostic Factors	Tumor Related	Host Related	Environment Related
Essential	T Category N category Extracapsular nodal extension Superior sulcus location Intrapulmonary metastasis	Weight loss Performance status	Resection margins Adequacy of mediastinal dissection
Additional	Histologic type Grade Vessel invasion Tumor size	Gender Age	Radiotherapy dose Adjuvant radiation
New and promising	Molecular/biologic markers	Quality of life Marital status	

Sources: NCCN Clinical Practice Guidelines in Oncology: Non-Small Cell Lung Cancer 2005. http:// www.nccn.org/professionals/physician_gls/PDF/nscl.pdf
Program in Evidence-Based Care: Practice Guidelines and Evidence Based Summaries Lung Cancer Site Group 2003. http://www.cancercare.on.ca/index_lungCancerguidelines.htm

Table 11.2 Prognostic Factors in Advanced[1] NSCLC

Prognostic Factors	Tumor Related	Host Related	Environment Related
Essential	Stage SVCO Solitary brain Solitary adrenal metastasis Number of sites	Weight loss Performance status	Chemoradio-therapy Chemotherapy
Additional	Number of metastatic sites Pleural effusion Liver metastases Hemoglobin LDH Albumin	Gender Symptom burden	
New and promising	Molecular/biologic markers	Quality of life Marital status Anxiety/depression	

[1]Locally advanced or metastatic.

Table 11.3 Prognostic Factors in SCLC

Prognostic Factors	Tumor Related	Host Related	Environment Related
Essential	Stage	Performance status Age Comorbidity	Chemotherapy Thoracic radiotherapy Prophylactic cranial RT
Additional	LDH Alkaline Phosphatase Cushing's syndrome M0 Mediastinal involvement M1 Number of sites bone or brain involvement WBC, Platelet count		
New and promising	Molecular/biologic markers		

Source: NCCN Clinical Practice Guidelines in Oncology: Non-Small Cell Lung Cancer 2005. http://www.nccn.org/professionals/physician_gls/PDF/sclc.pdf

References:

1. Cameron R, Loehrer Sr, Thomas CR Jr: Neoplasms of the Mediastinum: in DeVita VT HS, Rosenberg SA, (eds.): Cancer: Principles and Practice of Oncology. 7th ed. Philadelphia: Lippincott-Raven; 2005, pp. 845-860.

2. Brundage MD, Davies D, Mackillop WJ: Prognostic factors in non-small cell lung cancer: a decade of progress. *Chest* 122:1037-1057, 2002.

3. Solan MJ, Werner-Wasik M. Prognostic factors in non-small cell lung cancer. *Semin Surg Oncol* 21:64-73, 2003.

4. Brundage MD, Mackillop WJ: Lung Cancer, in Gospodarowicz MK HD, Hutter RVP, O'Sullivan B, et al. (eds.): Prognostic Factors in Cancer. 2nd ed. New York, Wiley-Liss; pp. 351-370, 2001.

5. Wittekind Ch, Henson DE, et al.: TNM Supplement. A commentary on uniform use. 3rd ed. New York, Wiley-Liss, 2003.

6. Arriagada R, Le Pechoux C, Pignon JP: Resected non-small cell lung cancer: need for adjuvant lymph node treatment? From hope to reality. *Lung Cancer* 42:S57-S64, 2003.

7. Sihoe AD, Yim AP: Lung cancer staging. *JSurg Res* 117:92-106, 2004.

8. Schrevens L, Larent N, Dooms C, et al.: The role of PET scan in diagnosis, staging, and management of non-small cell lung cancer. *Oncologist* 9:633-643, 2004.

9. Ukena D, Hellwig D: Value of FDG PET in the management of NSCLC. *Lung Cancer* 45:S75-S78, 2004.

10. O'Byrne KJ, Cox G, Swinson D, et al.: Towards a biological staging model for operable non-small cell lung cancer. *Lung Cancer* 34:S83-S89, 2001.

11. Kraut MJ, Vallieres E, Thomas CR Jr: Pancoast (superior sulcus) neoplasms. *Curr Probl Cancer* 27:81-104, 2003.

12. Fried DB, Morris DE, Poole C, et al.: Systematic review evaluating the timing of thoracic radiation therapy in combined modality therapy for limited-stage small-cell lung cancer. *J Clin Oncol* 22:4837-4845, 2004.

APPENDIX: PROGNOSTIC FACTORS IN LUNG CANCER – INFORMATION FROM THE IASLC INTERNATIONAL DATA BASE*

The IASLC Staging Project studied the impact of those prognostic factors, in addition to the anatomical extent of disease, for which data was available in the International data base. The findings have been reported in detail (1;2) and only a brief summary is included here.

Information available from clinically staged cases for which cTNM data was available.

Among the potentially useful prognostic variables for lung cancer survival, data for many were not available in the IASLC staging project database, such as those related to tumour biology or the role of fluoro-deoxy-glucose position emission tomography (FDG-PET) scanning. For this reason, the analysis was restricted to those variables for which enough information was available in a significant number of patients. These included clinical stage, expressed as TNM for non-small cell lung cancer (NSCLC) and limited disease (LD) versus extensive disease (ED) for small-cell lung cancer (SCLC), age, gender, performance status (PS) and histological cell type. For NSCLC, 12,428 cases with stage I-IV disease were assessable and for SCLC, 6,609 (3,739 with ED and 2,870 with LD). For smaller subsets of SCLC and advanced stage NSCLC, laboratory values were available on serum calcium, serum albumin, serum sodium, haemoglobin and white blood cell count (WBC).

a) For cases of NSCLC when prognostic factors were analysed by clinical stage, as proposed by the IASLC staging project, histology cell type was a significant prognostic factor for survival only in patients with stage IIIA,

---

Note: The Appendix published on pages 134-140 is reprinted with permssion from the Journal of Thoracic Oncology; *see refs. 1-3, page 140. Copyright International Association for the Study of Lung Cancer.*

while PS, gender and age were significant in all stages, but with a lower limit for age in advanced stages. Using recursive partitioning and amalgamation analysis (RPA) 4 groups with significantly different prognosis were identified: Group 1 with stage IA-IIA (any age and any PS); Group 2 with stage IIB/IIIA and PS 0-1 (any age); Group 3 with stage IIB/IIIA and PS 2 (any age) or with stage IIIB/IV and PS 0 (any age) or with stage IIIB/IV, age <81 years and PS 1; Group 4 with stage IIB/IIIA and PS 3-4 (any age) or with stage IIIB/IV and PS 2-4 (any age) or with stage IIIB/IV, PS 1 and age >80 years. The resulting amalgamated categories were applied to a survival analysis on the validation set of patients. Median survival times were respectively 53 months for group 1, 16 months for group 2, 8 months for group 3 and 3 months for group 4.

A total of 7,280 cases with advanced, stage IIIB or IV, NSCLC in the database had data on at least one of the following laboratory values in addition to the other prognostic factors (age, gender, PS): calcium (1,316 cases), albumin (1,887 cases), sodium (1,708 cases), haemoglobin (1,564 cases) and white blood cells (WBC) (2,126 cases). A Cox model was performed with each individual laboratory value and the other prognostic factors. The laboratory variables in advanced NSCLC appeared to be strong prognostic factors in a magnitude similar to PS while age and gender were weaker. In 537 patients, data was available on all of the five laboratory values. A multivariate model identified as strong significant prognostic factors ($p<0.001$) PS and WBC, followed by calcium ($p=0.0077$), albumin ($p=0.013$) and age ≥ 75 years ($p=0.0415$).

b) For cases of SCLC all variables tested (PS, extent of disease, gender and age) were found to be independent prognostic factors for survival. In patients with ED or LD the same independent prognostic factors (PS, gender and age) were identified as in NSCLC. Using RPA four groups with differing prognoses were identified : group 1 with LD, PS 0 and age <60 years or LD, PS 1-2 and age < 65 years; group 2 with LD, PS 1-2, age ≥ 65 years or female with ED, PS 0, and age < 65 years; group 3 females with ED, PS0 and age ≥ 65 years or males with ED, PS 0 or both genders with ED, PS 1, age < 70 years; group 4 with LD PS 3-4 or with ED, PS 1, age ≥ 70 years or with ED, PS 2-4. The resulting amalgamated categories were applied to a survival analysis in the validation set. Median survival times were respectively 17 months for group I, 12 months for group 2, 10 months for group 3 and 6 months for group 4.

A total of 6,609 cases with SCLC in the database had data on at least one of the following laboratory values in addition to the other prognostic factors (stage, age, gender, PS): calcium (1,849 cases), albumin (2,773 cases), sodium (2,390 cases), haemoglobin (1,487 cases) and white blood cells (WBC) (1,828 cases). A Cox model was performed with each individual laboratory value and the other prognostic factors. Two laboratory variables (sodium and albumin) appeared to be very significant prognostic factors in addition to stage, PS and gender. In 650 patients there was data available on all five laboratory values. A multivariate model identified albumin only, in addition to extent of disease and gender, as significant prognostic factors.

c) **Summary.** Our findings are summarised in Table 11.4. Many potentially useful prognostic variables were not investigated because of missing data or missing variables, inevitable in a retrospective database. Some could not be assessed because they had only recently been suggested, such as for those related to molecular biology or to the value of PET scanning. In regard to the role of molecular or biological markers in lung cancer, more than 5,000 articles have been published, often of varying methodological quality. The best evidence available in the literature at present on this subject has come from the meta-analyses summarised in Table 11.5. The estimate of the prognostic value of these variables reported in these studies is limited by the use of univariate analyses. The independent role of the prognostic factors identified in this study has to be confirmed in prospective studies. The prognostic value of the primary tumour SUV max (maximal standard uptake value) measured on FDG-PET has been assessed by a meta-analysis of the literature, undertaken by the European Lung Cancer Working Party evidence-based medicine committee for the IASLC staging project. This showed that SUV max is a strong prognostic factor for survival in a univariate analysis (3). This should be confirmed by a meta-analysis based on individual patient data allowing multivariate analysis to be performed which takes into account the prognostic factors identified in the present article.

The analysis of the database of the IASLC staging project identified important prognostic factors for survival in lung cancer patients in addition to clinical stage. Those factors were performance status, age and gender. In stage IIIA NSCLC, histological cell type appeared to be important. In advanced NSCLC some routine laboratory tests were found to be additional, significant factors. In SCLC, albumin was found to also an independent prognostic factor. Models were constructed using a recursive partitioning and amalgamation method for both NSCLC and SCLC. They allowed the identification of groups of patients with differing prognoses, taking into account clinical stage and PS and, to a lesser extent, age and gender. Although the results reported in this study were obtained in the largest series ever used for prognostic analysis in lung cancer, the prognostic variables and models found require to be confirmed by a prospective study, such as that already planned by the IASLC Lung Cancer Staging Project.

Table 11.4 Summary of the Prognostic Factors with a Grading as Following: ++++ and +++ = factors present in any model; ++ = factors significant in RPA and Cox models; + = factors significant in Cox models (or in a meta-analysis for SUVmax); +§ = biological factors significant in Cox models not taking into consideration other biological variables.

Variable	NSCLC	SCLC
Clinical Extentof Disease[#]	+ + + +	+ + + +
Performance status[°]	+ + + (≥ IIB only)	+ + +
Age	++ (≥ IIIB only)	+ +
Male gender	+	++
Squamous cell type	+ (IIIA only)	N/A
PET SUV_{max}	+	N/A
Calcium	+[*]	–
Albumin	+[*]	+
Sodium	+§[*]	+§
White blood cells	+[*]	–
Haemoglobin	+§ [*]	-

N/A = not applicable/not available.
Extent of disease by TNM stage for NSCLC and LD/ED for SCLC.
° performance status by Zubrod scale.
* Advanced stage IIIB/IV for NSCLC.

Information available from pathologically staged cases for which pTNM data was available.

Here we examined primarily a subset of those prognostic factors (cell type, age, and gender) in 9,137 pathologically staged I-IIIA NSCLC surgically managed cases in the IASLC data base, selecting from databases that distinguished the bronchioloalveolar carcinoma (BAC) subtype from the other adenocarcinomas as a separate category. The large number of cases and relatively homogenous group with respect to management (surgery as part of definitive treatment in all cases) allowed us to explore the prognostic impact of cell type in greater detail than has been possible in the analyses of single institution series or of population-based registries. In consideration of the potential for disproportionate representation of the different cell types within patient groups, particular care was taken to explore the relationship with respect to survival between stage, cell type, and gender.

The adenocarcinoma and squamous cell carcinoma histologies comprised the largest proportions of the study sample (36% and 49% respec-

Table 11.5 Meta-analysis Published on the Prognostic Value of Biological or Genetic Markers for Survival in Lung Cancer.

Biological Variable	Prognostic Factors
bcl-2	Favorable
TTF1	Adverse
Cox2	Adverse
EGFR	Adverse
ras	Adverse
Ki67	Adverse
HER2	Adverse
VEGF	Adverse
microvascular density	Adverse
p53	Adverse
aneuploidy	Adverse

tively). Squamous cell carcinomas predominated in stages II and III and were less frequently stage I (35%) as compared to the adenocarcinomas (46%). There were imbalances with respect to gender and histology. Among females, 55% were adenocarcinoma and 25% squamous cell. In contrast, the male cases were 30% adenocarcinoma and 57% squamous cell.

Survival was found to correlate with pathologic TNM category (IASLC proposals for TNM 7th edition) as expected, with median survival estimates ranging from 19 months for stage IIIA to 95 months for stage IA. For cell type across all stages combined, the BAC subtype has a median survival of 83 months, followed by adenocarcinoma, 45 months, versus 44 months for squamous cell carcinomas, 34 months for large cell, and 26 months for adenosquamous.

The following variables were considered in Cox proportional hazards regression analyses: pTNM stage grouping, age, gender, and histological cell type. Unadjusted analyses, in which each factor was considered independently, revealed significant differences between BAC and all other cell types, between males and females, and between patients 70 and older versus patients less than 70 years of age. In unadjusted analyses across all stages and both genders, the adenocarcinomas and squamous cell carcinomas did not have a significantly different prognosis. However, in a model including all factors, cell type, pathologic stage, gender, and age, squamous cell has a significant survival advantage over adenocarcinoma and large cell, suggesting that, all other things being equal, the squamous cell carcinoma histology carries a slightly better prognosis. There was no significant difference between large cell and adenocarcinoma, or between adenosquamous and any other non-BAC histology.

There was a small but statistically significant interaction between histology and gender. In females, there is no significant difference between squamous cell carcinomas and adenocarcinomas or between any other non-BAC histologies after adjusting for stage and other factors, although the survival estimates favoured the adenocarcinoma cases. There was, however, a significant survival advantage for squamous cell carcinoma over adenocarcinoma and large cell among males, and this appeared to be the source for the finding that there is a small survival advantage for squamous cell carcinomas over-all. Within stage groups, no differences were seen between any of the non-BAC histologies that reached significance, although the hazard ratios in the stage II and III categories favoured the squamous cell cases, and BAC had a significant survival advantage (P=<.0001) among the stage I cases only.

Stage, age, gender, and cell type were entered into a recursive partitioning and amalgamation (RPA) analysis to generate a survival tree of recursive splits on the dataset. Viewing only the splits that were statistically significant after accounting for multiple tests, stage, age, and gender remained as important variables. The most important factor overall is pTNM stage, and within stage categories, age is prognostic.

We concluded that for surgically managed pathologically staged I-IIIA NSCLC (according to the IASLC proposals for the 7th edition of TNM), age, gender, and to a lesser degree certain cell types, in addition to pTNM stage are all prognostic factors. Stage remains to be the most important factor, followed by age, and in early stage cases, gender. The cases classified as BAC in this dataset would have varied from pure non-invasive BAC to invasive adenocarcinoma with BAC components. Nevertheless, this category had a prognosis distinct from the other subtypes. Regarding a comparison of the two most common NSCLC lung cancer histologies, the squamous cell carcinomas may have a better prognosis than the non-BAC adenocarcinomas, particularly among males with early stage disease, but the question remains as to whether the undetected inclusion of the BAC subtype within the adenocarcinomas obscures what might otherwise be a survival advantage for squamous cells in females as well as males.

References:

(1) Sculier JP, Chansky K, Crowley JJ, Van Meerbeeck J, Goldstraw P, IASLC International Staging Project. The impact of additional prognostic factors on survival and their relationship with the Anatomical Extent of Disease as expressed by the 6th edition of the TNM Classification of Malignant Tumours and the proposals for the 7th edition. *J Thorac Oncol* 3, 457-466. 2008.

(2) Chansky K, Sculier JP, Crowley JJ, Giroux DJ, Van Meerbeeck J, Goldstraw P, et al. The IASLC Lung Cancer Staging Project: Prognostic Factors and Pathologic TNM Stage in Surgically Managed Non-Small Cell Lung Cancer. *J Thorac Oncol* 4, 792-801. 2009.

(3) Berghmans T, Dusart M, Paesmans M, Hossein-Foucher C, Buvat I, Castaigne C, et al. Primary tumor standardized uptake value (SUVmax) measured on fluorodeoxyglucose positron emission tomography (FDG-PET) is of prognostic value for survival in non-small cell lung cancer (NSCLC): a systematic review and meta-analysis (MA) by the European Lung Cancer Working Party for the IASLC Lung Cancer Staging Project. *J Thorac Oncol* 3, 6-12.2008.

MALIGNANT PLEURAL MESOTHELIOMA

Nirmal K. Veeramachaneni and Richard J. Battafarano

Approximately 2000-3000 cases of diffuse malignant pleural mesothelioma (DMPM) are diagnosed each year in the United States. While exposure to asbestos remains the leading risk factor for development of DMPM, 20% of patients have no prior history of asbestos exposure.[1] The natural history of DMPM is one of locoregional progression with development of distant metastasis. The presentation of the tumor is often insidious, and delay in diagnosis is common. Despite aggressive multimodality treatment, the median survival is poor ranging from 4-18 months.[1,2]

Mesotheliomas are classified into epithelial, sarcomatoid, desmoplastic, and biphasic types.[3] Epithelial type is the most common (50-57%) histology and is associated with the best prognosis. Biphasic (24-34%) and sarcomatoid histologies (16-19%) are associated with a poor prognosis, with essentially no 5-year survivors in the largest reported series. Desmoplastic mesothelioma, in which >50% of the tumor consists of dense hypocellular collagen, has a similarly poor prognosis with a median survival of 6 months. As such, some authors consider desmoplastic mesothelioma to be a variant of sarcomatoid mesothelioma. Accurate tissue diagnosis is essential because the prognosis is based heavily upon histologic typing.[4]

In order to obtain adequate tissue for pathologic examination, invasive measures, such as video assisted thoracoscopy, or open pleural biopsy, are required. Cervical mediastinoscopy provides access to the paratracheal and subcarinal lymph nodes for lymph node staging. Fine needle aspiration biopsies often do not yield adequate tissue to differentiate malignant pleural mesothelioma from metastatic adenocarcinoma to the pleura. The surgeon must be cognisant of the biopsy strategy, and orient the incisions to permit definitive resection of the biopsy site(s) at a later time. Combinations of computerized tomography (CT) and positron emission tomography (PET) imaging are useful in assessing locoregional and distant disease.[5,6] Magnetic resonance (MRI) is a useful adjunct to assess the degree of local involvement and suitability for resection.[7]

Combinations of surgery, radiation therapy, and chemotherapy have been attempted with varying success. Evidence is based mainly from nonrandomized studies with small sample sizes and over differing and lengthy time periods. In the setting of favorable histology, resectable disease and minimal comorbidities, complete surgical resection may be accomplished by extrapleural pneumonectomy.[8] A more limited resection, such as pleurectomy and decortication, may be offered if negative margins can be achieved.[9]

Adjuvant therapy using hyperthermic cisplatin-based chemotherapy at the time of pneumonectomy, photodynamic therapy to eradicate microscopic disease, and radiation treatment to the surgically resected field have been employed by various institutions with varying degrees of success.[10] Combination chemotherapy, particularly platinum containing regimens in nonsurgical candidates continues to be actively studied. The best available data regarding prognostic variables are from large series of patients treated with aggressive surgical resection,[8] as well as collective reviews of phase II chemotherapy trials.[11]

To identify those most likely to benefit from aggressive therapy, considerable effort has focused on developing a universally accepted staging system.[12] Initial efforts by Butchart and Sugarbaker defined stage by local tumor invasion and resected margins, but these systems did not provide adequate prognostic information due to limitations of imaging modalities. The most recent TNM classification is a modification of the International Mesothelioma Interest Group system, and differentiates tumors by tumor size, lymph node involvement, and the presence of metastatic disease.[13] These different systems clearly indicate that microscopically positive resection margins (Rl) confer a worse prognosis, as does the presence of involved subcarinal or mediastinal lymph nodes.[14] In many studies, no long-term survivors were reported in the presence of lymph node metastasis.[14,15] Due to the aggressive nature of this malignancy, careful patient selection is necessary both to identify those most likely to benefit from multimodality therapy, and to minimize treatment related morbidity and mortality.

MALIGNANT THYMOMA

Andrea Bezjak and David G. Payne

Tumors of the thymus are rare, accounting for 15% of mediastinal tumors. Most thymomas are slow growing tumors with a long natural history. Recurrences can be seen decades after seemingly successful initial treatment. These issues have management implications with a lack of high-quality evidence to guide practice. Most evidence is based on case series of often heterogenous patient groups who were treated with a variety of modalities over a prolonged period of time.[1]

Stage is the most important prognostic factor. The most frequently used staging classification for thymomas originally comes from Masaoka[2] with the proposed UICC TNM classification[3] using similar criteria. The Masaoka stage is based on the degree of invasion of thymoma into surrounding tissues, as determined by imaging and/or at the time of resection and subsequent histopathological examination. Recent reports detail the distribution of cases, and the associated rates of recurrence and survival.[4,5] Another essential prognostic factor is pathologic subtype of thymoma. A number of pathologic classifications have been proposed, starting with the Bernatz classification of spindle cell thymomas, lymphocytic thymomas (both associated with excellent survival rates), epithelial, and mixed-cell types (associated with poorer rates of survival). Subsequent Marino-Muller-Hermelink classification, based on the degree of differentiation of the malignant cell toward a pattern corresponding to the thymic cortex or medulla, was confirmed to be of prognostic significance,[6] with medullary, mixed, and well-differentiated organoid tumors being associated with early stage thymomas. Histology and the Masaoka stage were independent predictors for overall ($p < 0.05$) and disease-free survival ($p < 0.004$, $p < 0.0001$). The current histologic classification is one developed by the World Health Organization (WHO); studies support its prognostic significance with 5- and 10-year survival rates as follows: 100% for types A and AB thymomas, 100% and 86% for type B1, 85% and 85% for B2, and 51% and 38% for B3, respectively.[7] The WHO histologic type was correlated with invasion into neighboring organs, recurrence rate, disease free survival, and overall survival.[4]

The mainstay of treatment of thymomas is surgery. The role of radiation in stage II completely resected thymomas is controversial, based on up to 40% local recurrence rates historically with surgery alone. However, more recent series of surgery alone have documented excellent local control.[8,9] Stage III thymomas are usually resected, followed by postoperative radiotherapy to reduce the risk of local relapse; doses of 40-50 Gy are used for microscopic disease, and 50-60 Gy for gross disease. This results in high rates of local control in the mediastinum, although a risk of pleural, pericardial, or lung parenchymal relapse remains and it is not clear if that can be mitigated by adjuvant treatment. Some authors advocate preoperative radiation of unresectable thymomas, and prophylactic pericardial or hemithoracic radiation to prevent relapses in those areas, but this remains controversial. The role of debulking surgery in unresectable stage III thymomas or resection of primary or metastatic deposits in stage IV thymomas is also unclear.[10] Chemotherapy is most commonly used to treat metastatic and/or recurrent disease, using a single drug (e.g., cisplatinum, prednisone) or more often multidrug combination. No regimen is widely accepted as standard. There is increasing interest in the use of induction chemotherapy prior to surgery and radiotherapy in advanced stage unresectable tumors, aiming to render the tumor resectable, and/or reduce the volume of normal lung at risk for subsequent radiation injury. Only Phase II studies have been performed, using a variety of regimens, usually containing platinum.

The amount of postoperative residual disease is an important prognostic factor, with 95% 5-year survival rates for completely resected disease, compared to 50% with subtotal resection.[11] Another series reported a 93% 5-year survival of patients with stages III and IV completely resected thymomas, versus 64.4% for patients with the same stages but subtotally resected.[12]

Other factors, that are prognostic in some series include

- Presence of paraneoplastic syndrome: In some (particularly older) series, myasthenia gravis has been identified as an adverse prognostic factor, due to increased perioperative mortality, however, with improved supportive care, it may actually be a favorable factor as it leads to an earlier diagnosis.[13]
- Tumor size: worse survival for large thymomas (<10 vs. ≥10 cm), e.g., 97% versus 72% 5-year survival.[7]

There are some newer promising molecular prognostic factors. Epidermal growth factor receptor has been found to be expressed in 28/37 patients with invasive thymomas;[14] c-KIT expression was more common in thymic carcinomas;[15] this may provide a therapeutic option that targets these receptors. Stage IV thymomas were found to have much higher expressions of Cten mRNA, and its expression was correlated with evidence of tumor progression.[16] Cten mRNA likely plays a role in focal adhesion, cell motility, and/or migration. Human homolog of rad17 gene (Hrad17) mRNA, which is implicated in cell checkpoint control, was found to be expressed at significantly higher levels in invasive thymomas (stages II-IV) than in stage I thymomas, and it was not present in normal thymus tissue. Diploid tumors had a significantly higher probability of survival as compared to aneuploid tumors.[17]

Future studies of molecular targets may offer new avenues of therapeutic approaches in thymomas.

Table 11.7 Prognostic Factors in Thymoma

Prognostic Factors	Tumor Related	Host Related	Environment Related
Essential	Cell type Clinical stage Metastases		
Additional	Size Paraneoplastic syndrome	Performance status Age	Access to care
New and promising	Aneuploidy EGFR p53 cKIT Cten mRNA		

Sources: National Cancer Institute: Thymoma (PDQ®): Treatment Guidelines 2003. http://www.cancer. gov/cancertopics/pdq/treatment/malignant-thymoma/healthprofessional/ British Columbia Cancer Agency Cancer Management Guidelines: Thymoma 2001. http://www.bccancer.bc.ca/HPI/CancerManagementGuidelines/Lung/Thymoma/default.htm

References:

1. Payne D: Malignant Thymoma: in Gospodarowicz MK, Henson DE, Hutter RVP, et al. (eds.), *Prognostic Factors in Cancer*. 2nd ed., New York, Wiley-Liss, 2001, pp. 387-398.

2. Rena O, Papalia E, Maggi G, et al: World Health Organization histologic classification: an independent prognostic factor in resected thymomas. *Lung Cancer* 50:59-66, 2005.

3. Wittekind Ch, Henson DE, et al: *TNM Supplement. A commentary on uniform use*. 3rd ed. New York, Wiley-Liss, 2003.

4. Kondo K, Yoshizawa K, Tsuyuguchi M, et al: WHO histologic classification is a prognostic indicator in thymoma. *Ann Thorac Surg* 77: 1183-1188, 2004.

5. Sonobe M, Nakagawa M, Ichinose M, et al: Thymoma: analysis of prognostic factors. *Jpn J Thor Cardiovasc Surg* 49:35-41, 2001.

6. Lardinois D, Rechsteiner R, Lang RH, et al. Prognostic relevance of Masaoka and Muller-Hermelink classification in patients with thymic tumors. *Ann Thorac Surg* 69:1550-1555, 2000.

7. Nakagawa K, Asamura H, Matsuno Y, et al. Thymoma: a clinicopathologic study based on the new World Health Organization classification. *J Thorac Cardiovasc Surg* 126:1134-1140, 2003.

8. Mangi AA, Wright CD, Allan JS, et al.: Adjuvant radiation therapy for stage II thymoma. *Ann Thorac Surg* 74:1033-1037, 2002.

9. Singhal S, Shrager JB, Rosenthal DI, et al.: Comparison of stages I-II thymoma treated by complete resection with or without adjuvant radiation. *Ann Thorac Surg* 76:1635-1641, discussion 1641-1642, 2003.

10. Zhu G, He S, Fu X, et al.: Radiotherapy and prognostic factors for thymoma: a retrospective study of 175 patients. *Int J Radiat Oncol Biol Phys* 60: 1113-1119, 2004.

11. Moore KH, McKenzie PR, Kennedy CW, et al.: Thymoma: trends over time. *Ann Thorac Surg* 72:203-207, 2001.

12. Kondo K, Monden Y: Therapy for thymic epithelial tumors: a clinical study of 1,320 patients from Japan. *Ann Thorac Surg* 76:878-884; discussion 884-875, 2003.

13. de Perrot M, Liu J, Bril V, et al.: Prognostic significance of thymomas in patients with myasthenia gravis. *Ann Thorac Surg* 74: 1658-1662, 2002.

14. Henley JD, Koukoulis GK, Loehrer PJ Sr: Epidermal growth factor receptor expression in invasive thymoma. *J Cancer Res Clin Oncol* 128: 167-170, 2002.

15. Henley JD, Cummings OW, Loehrer PJ Sr: Tyrosine kinase receptor expression in thymomas. *J Cancer Res Clin Oncol* 130:222-224, 2004.

16. Sasaki H, Yukiue H, Kobayashi Y, et al.: Cten mRNA expression is correlated with tumor progression in thymoma. *Tumour Biol* 24:271-274, 2003.

17. Gawrychowski J, Rokicki M, Gabriel A, et al.: Thymoma-the usefulness of some prognostic factors for diagnosis and surgical treatment. *Eur J Surg Oncol* 26:203-208, 2000.

Editor's Note: *Those involved in the development of the TNM classification are grateful to colleagues who post questions on the UICC TNM Helpdesk regarding difficult staging scenaria that arise in clinical practice. Many such questions raise fundamental issues regarding stage classification which cannot be answered from available data. In giving advice one often has to fall back on the General Principles of the TNM classification, which become strengthened, and occasionally modified, by such interrogation. To ensure uniformity in the application of TNM the responses are collated for future reference. We include here some "Frequently Asked Questions" to help the reader and stimulate future debate.*

Acknowledgement: *Used with the permission of the International Union Against Cancer (UICC), Geneva, Switzerland. The original source for this material is the TNM Supplement: A Commentary on Uniform Use, 4th Edition (2009) published by John Wiley & Sons Ltd, www.wiley.com.*

CHAPTER 12 | Frequently Asked Questions

The following are a selection of frequently asked questions that have been chosen to illustrate some of the more common problems referred to the TNM Helpdesk.

Q How does one classify a patient with a tumour obstructing the right main bronchus, in which the resultant collapse/consolidation of the middle and lower lobes obscures the margins of the tumour and one cannot assess its size?

A The features described suggest that the tumour is at least T2 but one cannot assess size to determine if it is T2a, T2b or T3. One should apply General Rule 4 in such circumstances. This states that "If there is doubt concerning the correct T, N or M category to which a particular case should be allotted, then the lower (i.e. less advanced)category should be chosen. This will be reflected in the stage grouping". This case should be classified as cT2a and if node negative is stage IB.

Q In the clinical staging of lung cancer: Should one measure the size of the tumour on the CT scan using the lung "window" or the mediastinal "window" settings?

A   One should perform the measurement on the "window" settings that in your institution give the most accurate assessment of tumour size. A diagnostic radiologist would be able to indicate which is the "window" giving the most accurate evaluation in your institution.

Q   How should one classify a patient with a 4cm spiculated lesion in the left lower lobe, and a 2cm lesion in the right upper lobe? A needle biopsy from the left lesion confirms adenocarcinoma. On PET scan there is high uptake in both of the lung lesions but no uptake elsewhere in the hilum, mediastinum or at distant sites. Does one need to biopsy the right lesion to confirm that it is of different cell type?

A   Whether or not a needle biopsy of the right lung lesion should be undertaken in this case depends upon whether the treatment approach proposed by the multi-disciplinary team would be influenced by the differing interpretations of the classification on the evidence so far available. This case could be classified as a) cT2a N0 M1a, stage IV or b) if shown to be synchronous primary tumours should be classified under General rule 5 which states that "in the case of multiple simultaneous tumours in one organ (the 2 lungs are considered to be a single organ for these purposes), the tumour with the highest T category should be classified and the multiplicity or the number of tumours should be indicated in parenthesis." This case could therefore be classified under b) as cT2a(m) N0 M0 or cT2a(2) N0 M0, stage IB. If treatment decisions would be influenced by knowing the cell type of the right-sided lesion, which might show a different cell type or provide morphological, immunohistochemical or molecular differences suggesting that the tumours are different sub-types of the same cell type, then a needle biopsy of the right-sided tumour would be justified for staging purposes.

Q   How should one classify a case in which an undifferentiated carcinoma of the left upper lobe is infiltrating the soft tissues of the chest wall. There is a positive lymph node adjacent to the chest wall lesion and no intrathoracic node involvement. Is this pM1 or pN1 if one considers the soft tissue as an infiltrated organ and the local node as regional node?

A   In answering this question one has to assume that clinical and pathological features have excluded this tumour being a soft-tissue primary (sarcoma) or a breast carcinoma. If this is so then the supplement advises: "In rare cases, one finds no metastases in the regional lymph nodes, but only in lymph nodes that drain an adjacent organ directly invaded by the primary tumour. The lymph nodes of the invaded site are considered as those of the primary site for N classification." Lymph nodes in the soft tissues of the chest wall nodes are not considered "regional" lymph nodes in lung cancer and hence the classification to be applied should be "pM1b".

Q A case of lung cancer is classified on clinical/pre-treatment assessment as cN0 or cN1. At surgery it is deemed to be irresectable because of extensive mediastinal invasion by the primary tumour. The pathologist can only confirm that resected/sampled mediastinal nodes from stations 4 and 7 are clear of disease. Should this case be classified as pNX, pN0 or pN1 ?

A The TNM classification sets prerequisites for the number and distribution of lymph nodes that are required to be examined histologically to establish the pN category. In lung cancer these prerequisites are:"Histological examination of hilar and mediastinal lymphadenectomy specimen(s) will ordinarily include 6 or more lymph nodes/stations. Three of these nodes/stations should be mediastinal, including the sub-carinal nodes (#7) and three from N1 nodes/stations." However, if all the lymph nodes examined are negative, but the number or distribution of the lymph nodes recommended to be ordinarily examined is not met, classify as pN0. The combination of pT4 pN0 cM0 would not fulfill the criteria necessary to establish a pathological stage and this case should be classified as clinical stage IIIA.

Q A patient underwent a wedge resection of the right upper lobe for a pT1N0M0 adenocarcinoma. Six months later a further tumour was discovered in the right upper lobe and the patient underwent completion upper lobectomy. The pathological examination of the surgical specimen showed that the new lesion was a metastasis within an intrapulmonary lymph node, and lymph node tissue was clearly seen with a capsule at the periphery of the new tumour. How should one classify this case?

A This should be classified as recurrent tumour in a lymph node and not as a new primary. It would be appropriate to classify this as rpT0 pN1 pM0.

Q A patient underwent right upper lobectomy with systematic nodal dissection. Pathological examination showed a pT1 adenocarcinoma and confirmed that the requirements for a full pathological examination of the lymph nodes had been met. We confirmed involvement of the interlobar lymph node station (#12) with no other deposits in N1 and N2 stations, except for isolated tumour cells (ITC) in a paratracheal station (# R4). Should we classify this case as pN1, pN0(i+) or pN2(i+)?

A The supplement only considers ITC as a sub-category of the pN0classification. Unfortunately if one assigned the category of pN0(i+) or created a new one of pN2(i+) the irrefutable evidence of pN1 disease would be obscured. We can only suggest that the case be classified as pN1.

Q Our surgeon undertook right upper lobectomy and resection of the fused apical segment of the right lower lobe in a patient following induction chemotherapy. Macroscopically the tumour is 3.5 cms in size and appears to involve the attached segment. However, on microscopy I cannot identify the visceral pleura of the oblique fissure to confirm invasion. How should one classify this case?

A The use of an elastin stain may facilitate the identification of the visceral pleura (see pp. 86-87). However, direct invasion of an adjacent lobe, even when the fissure is deficient and there is no pleural separation at the point of invasion is classified at T2. This case should be classified as ypT2a.

Q On pathological examination of a resection specimen there is a 6 cm tumour with direct invasion into hilar fat. Is hilar fat considered evidence of mediastinal invasion or does this qualify as invasion of the mediastinal pleura? Is this categorized as pT2b, pT3 or pT4?

A Invasion of hilar fat is not included in any of the present T descriptors and we have no data on which to give advice. In this case there needs to be a dialogue between the surgeon and the pathologist. If the surgeon undertook a lobectomy and was certain that the resection margins were clear of disease, and if the pathologists confirms an R0 resection, then one can be reasonably sure that the "hilar" fat is truly hilar and one could assign the pT2b category to this case. If a pneumonectomy had been performed then there would be real concern that the "hilar" fat is really "mediastinal" fat. If the discussion between the patholo-gist and the surgeon concluded that this was the case then the pT4 cat-egory should be assigned. Further discussions would no doubt centre on whether this constituted an R1 resection!

Q Pathological examination of a resection specimen has shown a 2.5 cm peripheral adenocarcinoma which involves the visceral pleura but does not extend through to the superficial surface of the pleura. Should this be classified as pT1b or pT2?

A Invasion of the visceral pleura is a T2 descriptor and is defined as "invasion beyond the elastic layer including invasion to the visceral pleural surface" The use of elastic stains is recommended when this feature is not clear on evaluation of H&E sections (see p X). If in this case the invasion extends beyond the elastic lamina the case should be classified as pT2a.

Q Clinical classification suggested that our patient had a T2 N2 M0 NSCLC. Pre-operative biopsy of ipsilateral medistinal nodes confirmed N2 disease and thoracotomy was not undertaken. Should this case be classified as cN2 or pN2? Should this case now be assigned a patho-logical stage?

A Microscopical confirmation of the nodal disease would allow this to be classified as pN2. However, to be designated a pathological stage the primary tumour must also have been confirmed on biopsy to establish the pT category.

⊃ **Advice on further questions may be obtained from the TNM Helpdesk by accessing the TNM Classification of Malignant Tumours page at the UICC website www.uicc.org.**

2007 be included in the prospective data base. These will include "atypical" carcinoid tumours, "typical" carcinoid tumours with unusual features such as nodal or distant metastases and large cell neuroendocrine carcinomas. A collaboration between the International Mesothelioma Interest Group and the IASLC, established at another IASLC workshop in London, in 2009, will ensure that cases of mesothelioma treated by all modalities of care from around the world will also be prospectively accrued and the proposals that emanate from this analysis will be incorporated within future IASLC proposals for revision of the TNM classification of Thoracic tumours.

Experience with the retrospective phase of the IASLC Staging Protect helped define the data elements required in the prospective phase. Baseline data will be captured at the time a decision is made as to first-line treatment of newly diagnosed lung cancer confirmed by histology or cytology, and will include patient characteristics, baseline laboratory values, treatment modalities, TNM stage and all supporting evidence. All patients will be followed for survival.

Data on patient characteristics include date of birth, race, sex, smoking history, weight loss, performance status, height, weight, and specific comorbid factors needed to calculate the Colinet score for each patient: tobacco consumption, renal insufficiency, respiratory comorbidity, cardiovascular comorbidity, neoplastic comorbidity, and alcoholism. Data will also be collected on the date of entry to clinical trials, if applicable, the method of disease detection, whether diagnosis was based on cytology and/or histology, the location of the primary tumour, the degree of differentiation, and histologic type. In the case of small-cell lung cancer (SCLC), information will be collected on the presence of paraneoplastic syndromes, such as the syndrome of inappropriate secretion of antidiuretic hormone (SIADH), ectopic adrenocorticotrophic hormone (ACTH), and the myasthenic syndrome.

Baseline laboratory parameters include LDH, haemoglobin, calcium, alkaline phosphatase, sodium, white cell count, neutrophil count, platelet count, and albumin, including the upper and lower limits of normal for each laboratory. Other prognostic factors of interest include the maximum Standardized Uptake Value (SUV max) on the initial Positron Emission Tomographic scan (PET), at the primary tumour site as well as at sites of nodal uptake, and pulmonary function tests.

Data collection on clinical/evaluative cTNM, and if appropriate post-surgical pTNM, will be sufficiently detailed to allow an assessment of the validity of all of the T, N, and M descriptors, with special attention to those that could not be validated in the retrospective database, as well as those not yet incorporated in the TNM classification. The means by which each category was assessed will be collected to provide an assessment of "classificatory certainty", the under-utilised "C" factor in the TNM classification. If resection of the primary was attempted, data will also be collected on the date of surgery and the outcome, in terms of the completeness of resection, classified according to the IASLC proposals within the 7th edition of TNM(3). Details will be collected on the timing and dose of chemo/radiotherapy, whether used in the adjuvant or induction setting or as primary treatment..

The intended objectives for each T, N, and M category, and other aspects of the study, are given in Table 13.1.

Table 13.1 Study Objectives

Component	Objective
T	a) Assess the prognostic impact of tumour size. b) Assess the classification capacity of each descriptor defining T-status. c) Study new conditions not included in the present T (e.g., differences between parietal pleura invasion and rib invasion).

N	a) Assess the prognostic impact of N-status.
	 b) Explore the prognostic impact of involved lymph node "zones" within N1 and N2 categories.
	 c) Assess the prognostic impact of:
	    i. Nodal extent (single vs multiple station involvement in N1 and N2 locations),
	    ii. Nodal size, i.e. the largest involved node within the relevant N category, and
	    iii. Individual nodes being involved in each nodal category.
	 d) Assess the prognostic impact of extracapsular extension.
	 e) Assess the prognostic impact of the N3 nodal location, i.e. contralateral mediastinum, ipsilateral or contralateral supraclavicular fossa.

M	a) Assess the prognostic impact of M-status, especially those descriptors now included within the new category of M1a proposed by the IASLC for the 7th edition.
	 b) Assess the prognostic impact of:
	    i. Single metastasis in a single organ
	    ii. Multiple metastases in a single organ, and
	    iii. Multiple metastases in several organs.

Other	a) Assess the prognostic impact of histologic type and grade. b) Assess the reliability of staging methods utilized in clinical staging (for those tumours with pre-treatment and post-surgical classification). c) Assess the prognostic impact of complete, incomplete, and uncertain resections, according to the proposed definitions of the IASLC. d) Assess the prognostic impact of clinical factors, including co-morbidity and pulmonary function tests. e) Assess the prognostic impact of maximum standard uptake value (SUV max), at the primary site and in any positive nodal sites, for those patients with positron emission tomography (PET) scans in the pre-treatment staging.

References:

(1) Giroux DJ, Rami-Porta R, Chansky K, Crowley JJ, Groome PA, Postmus PE, et al. The IASLC Lung Cancer Staging Project: Data Elements for the Prospective Project. *J Thorac Oncol.* In press 2009.

(2) Lim E, Goldstraw P, Nicholson AG, Travis WD, Jett JR, Ferolla P, et al. Proceedings of the IASLC International Workshop on Advances in Neuroendocrine Tumors 2007. *J Thorac Oncol* 3, 1194-1201. 2008.

(3) Rami-Porta R, Wittekind C, Goldstraw P. Complete resection in lung cancer surgery:proposed definition. *Lung Cancer* 49, 25-33. 2005.

Any institution or individual considering participation in the prospective phase of the IASLC Staging Project may view the protocol at:

www.iaslc.org/links.asp

INDEX